Daisy,

Just wanted to thank you and let you know
I appreciate you for trusting us to help you
be the best you.
I'm proud of how far you have come!

I'm looking forward to seeing all you can
achieve!

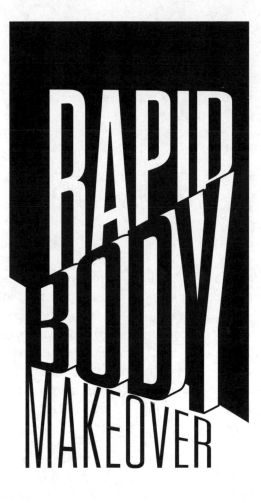

Published by CelebrityPress®, Orlando, FL

CelebrityPress® is a registered trademark

Printed in the United States of America.

ISBN: 978-0-9912143-7-2
LCCN: 2014941000

This publication is designed to provide accurate and authoritative information with regard to the subject matter covered. It is sold with the understanding that the publisher is not engaged in rendering legal, accounting, or other professional advice. If legal advice or other expert assistance is required, the services of a competent professional should be sought. The opinions expressed by the authors in this book are not endorsed by Celebrity Press® and are the sole responsibility of the authors rendering the opinion.

Most CelebrityPress® titles are available at special quantity discounts for bulk purchases for sales promotions, premiums, fundraising, and educational use. Special versions or book excerpts can also be created to fit specific needs.

For more information, please write:
CelebrityPress®
520 N. Orlando Ave, #2
Winter Park, FL 32789
or call 1.877.261.4930

Visit us online at: www.CelebrityPressPublishing.com

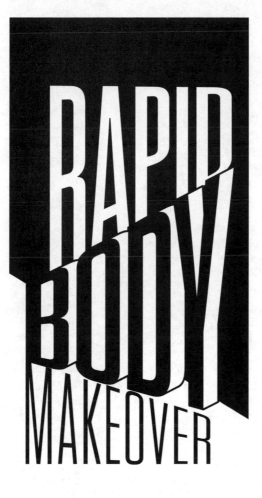

CELEBRITY PRESS®
Winter Park, Florida

CONTENTS

CHAPTER 1

MENTAL AND EMOTIONAL OPTIMIZATION FOR YOUR RAPID BODY *MAKEOVER*

BY JOHN SPENCER ELLIS

What would you say if I told you that the physical transformation was the *least* important aspect of a *rapid body makeover*?

After working as both a personal trainer and personal development coach for a variety of clients across the globe, I can confidently say that the mental aspect of any makeover is the true key to genuine success. It is required – nothing optional about it – for lasting change. I have seen physically powerful people with weak mental and emotional dedication fail miserably at reaching their goals, and I have seen many others with undeveloped biceps and no athletic experience rapidly and powerfully change their bodies because they had a smart and determined mindset.

Changing your body will **always** entail changing your mental and emotional perspective as well. It's all connected. When you optimize these aspects of your life, your *rapid body makeover* will also be a *lifelong* body makeover, rather than just a quick fix or short-term change. If you have ever tried a crash or fad diet, you were likely only focusing on the physical change, rather than your whole self, which is why the results were likely so difficult to maintain. When you bring your body and mind, thoughts and emotions together, it's a brand new ball game. It's a new mindset and a new definition of who you are.

With that said, you can use your thoughts and emotions to optimize your rapid body makeover or to sabotage it.

THE MIND AND BODY CONNECTION

How do your mental and emotional states affect your body?

Think about how your body feels when you are sad or angry or surprised or fascinated. When you are sad, you might actually feel a physical ache in your chest or a dull pain in your head. Likewise, when you are exhilarated, you might enjoy a sudden burst of energy or feel tingly all over. Our emotions and thoughts play a large role in how our body feels and, ultimately, how it performs and responds to any makeover technique.

The same goes for our thoughts. Say the following out loud, in a quiet, ashamed voice: "I am weak." And then try this in a confident and bold voice: "I am strong." Just three words and the thoughts and intention that accompany them can change how your body feels and reacts, which is why it is so important to focus on the positive. Many of us have little voices in our heads that are constantly undermining our efforts.

Yogis have recognized and utilized the mind-body connection for centuries, and more coaches and athletes are acknowledging the importance of the whole package – of everything working in unison to help you achieve your goal, whether it's winning a race, healing an injury, losing weight or making over your body from the inside out.

When your mind and body perform as a team, rather than as combatants in a duel, they will both get that much stronger. When you believe that you can achieve a goal or change your body, your body will quickly respond to that positive reinforcement. Likewise, if you doubt yourself every step of the way, your body will hear that message loud and clear and offer up proof in poor results.

Since the mind has such a profound effect on the body, it is very important to listen to what it has to say. And if you don't like what you are currently hearing, it is also important to make a change.

MENTAL AND EMOTIONAL MAKEOVERS

Do you need a mental or emotional makeover just as much as a *rapid body makeover*?

If you constantly say "no, I can't do that," if you constantly put yourself in last place, or if you constantly judge yourself and others, then the answer to that question is a definite "yes."

Mental and emotional optimization involves taking a good, long look at your thoughts and emotions so that you can understand how they affect the rest of your life.

Try the following exercise for one day:

- Whether on your tablet, smart phone or a simple piece of paper, write down the emotions that you feel at various times of day. This can be "depressed" at 6 a.m., "weary" at 10 a.m., "happy" at 5 p.m. and so on.

- Likewise, notice what you were doing when you were feeling those emotions. If the depressed feelings are associated with waking up and going to work, note that. If you feel sluggish when you drink your fourth energy drink, note that as well.

- At the end of the day, take just five minutes to write down any words that come to mind as to how you feel about yourself (smart, scared, weak, silly, interested, etc.).

When you take a look at the results, it likely won't take long for you to determine just how you feel about yourself and how you think about yourself and your life as a whole. If you have a lot of optimistic observations recorded, then you are on track for a successful rapid body makeover; your body will respond to the positive reinforcement it regularly receives. If the results are less enthusiastic than you would like, then you know that it is time to make a change for the better. That recognition is the first step in your makeover.

DECIDE TO MAKE A CHANGE

While the seasons and the weather will change from month to month without much input from us, as humans, we have to make the conscious decision to change. No one else can do it for us. We have to decide to go back to school for a master's degree, decide to change career paths, decide to move to a new city or new neighborhood, decide to start or end a relationship, decide to change our bodies without the power of our thoughts and emotions. It is a mindset that starts with making an intentional decision.

This mindset also involves identifying yourself as a well or fit person rather than as someone who is weak, unwell or unworthy of great health and a great life. It comes from within. Someone who "goes on a diet" or "starts a program" has a default setting of short-term focus and short-lived results. A diet or program is something that is external, it is not intrinsic to who you are as a fit person. A healthy person simply lives a good life because it's who they are and what they believe in, rather than what they do for a short period of time. When you redefine yourself, you will, in turn, redefine your life for the better. You will also want to ensure that you have the very best people in your life, the right people who have already adopted this philosophy on life. You should literally fire the people from your life who will sabotage your healthy efforts and who are not willing to support you along the way. While this isn't easy, it will make a big difference in your ultimate success and happiness.

Now that you have decided to make a change, just what do you want to change? Your arms, your confidence, your relationship, your heart and lungs, your energy level, your overall health?

Once you have determined *what* you want to change and why you want to change, then you can start progressing confidently in that direction.

You may have several aspects of your life, mindset and body that you want to update. While it is ok to have multiple goals, you shouldn't try to change everything all at once. When you can focus in on what you want most, you will have a better chance of achieving one or two specific goals, rather than going after dozens of general ones without a lot of focus.

It may sound cheesy, but there is no better day to decide to make a change than today. Stop putting yourself off, stop putting yourself second, stop saying "maybe tomorrow…" You can decide to use the power of your thoughts and emotions to strengthen, open, empower and change your body and your life. It's the decision that only you can make and now is the perfect time to make it.

THE MIND AND BODY IN MOTION

Whether you are watching a successful Olympic athlete on TV or witnessing your older sister overcome a significant health challenge, it is the same principle in action. The mind and body can work together for the better – or for the worse. If you are struggling to get your mind and body on the same page, think of examples of people who serve to inspire you and motivate you. What do you think makes them determined and successful? How can you bring those qualities into your life?

Likewise, take the time to notice when your mind and body are working in unison and when they aren't. What feels different? What do you like about the former? Ultimately, you will be able to inspire yourself (and others), but seeking powerful examples in the beginning can be both encouraging and motivating. Likewise, getting at your own motivations provides powerful information that you can use in your *rapid body makeover*.

In addition, as you put your makeover plan in motion, motion itself can really be your friend. A long walk can help clear your head and a yoga class can help you breathe a little easier. Exercise releases feel-good endorphins that can give you a confidence and energy boost for hours to come. The more you move and the stronger you get, the more you will feel the myriad benefits in your mind and your body and the more you will change your life for the better.

MAKE WELLNESS A PART OF EVERY DAY

As we have discussed, mental, physical and emotional health are not just something you do for the short term. Rather, they are part of an overall healthy and happy life. With that in mind, you should make wellness a part of every single day, every single thought and every single action.

So when you hop on your bike, get ready to Zumba or pick up some dumbbells, it's not just a workout – it's who you are. When you prepare your lunches for the week or meet a friend for brunch on the weekend, it's not just a meal – it's who you are. It's all about how you sleep, eat, exercise, interact, think, move and what you say to yourself and to others.

When wellness becomes a ritual and a habit and a true part of every single day, when it is ingrained in your life and into everything you think, say and do, your overall health will benefit greatly. Sooner than later, you won't even have to think about being healthy because good habits, decisions and actions will be a natural part of your happy, healthy life.

RECORD YOUR PROGRESS

Just like an accountant keeps track of cash flow in and out of a business and a receptionist keeps track of upcoming client appointments, recording your progress will help you track your ups and downs and your overall progress. It will keep you both honest and aware.

You can use a variety of programs and apps that are designed to record everything from food to exercise to sleep, or you can create your own journal or log. The format itself is less important than the regularity and consistency of the effort. One bad day can quickly spiral into one bad week or one bad month, so following your progress with a watchful eye will let you know when you need to refocus and redouble your efforts and commitment. Tracking your progress is all about accountability.

Over time, you can also note key areas of challenge, such as Tuesday "happy hours" with your coworkers or spending time with friends who don't really support your desire to make a change, giving you the opportunity to update your lifestyle as needed. Recording your progress will also let you know when you have reached your goal, so that you can celebrate your success and celebrate yourself, and perhaps make plans for that next goal.

STAYING ON TRACK AND STAYING MOTIVATED

If you have ever lost weight, increased muscle mass, trained for an event or achieved another physical goal, then you may know that the hard part comes next: maintenance and staying motivated.

At this point, it's less about calories and fat grams, time spent at the gym and time spent reading about healthy living and more about your mindset. If you believe you can maintain your makeover, you will. It really is that simple. It's all about who you are on the inside and what you believe you are capable of. I have witnessed many clients undergo *rapid body makeovers* and maintain their results for years and decades to come through the power of positive self-talk, strong support circles, and belief in themselves and their efforts.

Here are my top tips for staying on track after you have reached your rapid body makeover goal:

- **Be social.** If you share your goal, progress and achievements with friends in person or on social media, you will be more likely to remain accountable. Maybe you have a workout buddy who you discuss your ongoing challenges with or maybe you keep a blog about the physical, mental and emotional ups and downs of your makeover – this is all about letting others who can encourage you understand where you are at. These people can encourage you and remind you of your goals and progress.

- **Be smart.** Once you have achieved a goal, yes, it is ok to give yourself a break on occasion. This might mean enjoying a strawberry ice cream cone every Sunday afternoon, taking a Pilates class instead of a kickboxing class or allowing yourself to enjoy a one-week vacation without conditions. But it does not mean that you let go of your mindset, your decision to change and your pride in your results. Be smart about staying on track and you won't have to start this process all over again next year. Remember who you are.

- **Be honest.** Are there things that you still need to work on? Maybe you need to find a sports therapist to talk to about ongoing body issues or find a training partner who has the ability to further motivate and challenge you. Honestly assess where you are at and where you still want to go and make sure you do this on a regular basis.

- **Be kind.** We are all pretty good at beating ourselves up and knocking ourselves down, but we are not always as great about complimenting and appreciating ourselves. And that is definitely part of the mental-emotional-physical connection. Look in the mirror, smile and appreciate your body and your mind and your self. Take time to mentally and physically celebrate your success and to be kind to yourself and the others who have supported you in your journey.

- **Be aware.** While there will be people around you who are absolutely thrilled at your *rapid body makeover*, there will also be others who will be jealous of all you have accomplished or worried that it means that you're leaving them behind. Make sure you spend time with the people who build you up and appreciate you for who you are. Again, just like a smart manager fires an employee who is trying to sabotage a business' efforts, you should also fire any fake friends who won't support you 100 percent of the way.

- **Be consistent.** Consistency likely got you to where you are and it will help keep you there – or even take you further. Be consistent in focusing on the positive, recording your progress, believing in yourself, making wellness a part of every day and moving forward with confidence.

- **Be accountable to yourself.** At the end of the day, you are the one who has achieved a *rapid body makeover*, who has overcome challenges and who is responsible for whatever is next. When you are accountable to yourself, you can't go wrong.

POSITIVE, LASTING CHANGE FOR THE BETTER

Making a positive and lasting change mentally, emotionally and physically is a really big deal. Many people have good intentions, but not everyone understands how important it is to optimize your mindset for real success. If you watch any weight-loss reality TV, you can see the light bulb turn on for the contestants who get it (and who often achieve real long-term success in their weight-loss goals and in their lives) and the ones who resist this notion that the mind and body are really connected.

Mental and emotional optimization will fuel your *rapid body makeover*, your long-term maintenance and your self-confidence. Working together, the mind and body are incredibly powerful.

When you harness the power of the mind-body connection and make a commitment to maintaining your results and believing in yourself, you will truly be unstoppable.

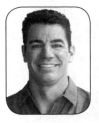

About John

Each week, over one million people enjoy a fitness and personal development program John created. He is the CEO of the National Exercise & Sports Trainers Association, Spencer Institute for Life Coaching, International Triathlon Coaching Association, MMA Conditioning Association, Get America Fit Foundation and Wexford University. He also created Adventure Boot Camp. He's a 2x Amazon #1 best-selling author, award-winning filmmaker and Personal Trainer Hall of Fame inductee. John competed in the Ironman triathlon and Brazilian Jiu Jitsu World Championships.

Dr. John Spencer Ellis holds degrees in health science, business, marketing and education. He has created over 500,000 jobs around the world. John helps fitness and coaching professionals become successful through education and dynamic marketing.

http://www.johnspencerellis.com

CHAPTER 2

RELEASING THE BRAKES — WHY 'JUST DO IT' THINKING WON'T GET YOU WHAT YOU WANT

BY DAX MOY

How many times have you started a new diet or exercise plan with the best of intentions and resolutions and promising yourself that, 'this time I WILL do this!' only to find that after only a few days (or even hours!) that all of your progress comes to a screeching halt…that your willpower crumbles to dust and that the very things that you promised yourself you wouldn't do are now being done…in supersize?

If you're anything like most people, the answer will be 'HUNDREDS of times' – right?

It's kind of strange when you think about it. On the one hand, we all tell ourselves that losing fat and getting into amazing shape is super-important to our health and happiness; yet whenever we're asked to prove just how important it really is by being committed and diligent in our efforts, we find it almost impossible to go the distance on our promises.

Why is that?

That's a question I used to ask myself all the time when I first set out on my personal training and coaching career. I'd meet people who would often literally burst into tears in my consulting room – because they were so overcome with pain and emotion as they told me "This MUST change!" and "I'm willing to do ANYTHING it takes to get things right this time" and "I simply cannot take living like this any longer!"

It was seriously moving stuff, and I, of course, believed every word of it. Why wouldn't I? After all, THEY believed every word of it too.

They really and truly believed that 'this time, this ONE time, I'm going to damned-well do this,' yet mere days later (or as much as a week or so for the *really* motivated ones) the first cracks would appear in their resolution and willpower.

One missed workout would become two, two would become three and before they knew what was happening, they were back to not working out at all. Same with nutrition and diet as the 'just one won't hurt' mentality asserted itself and was once again proven wrong. One cookie became two, two became a packet and a packet became licence to say, *"Well, now that I've messed up again, what's the point of carrying on?"*

As a trainer and a coach, this left me floating between genuine confusion about what was going on and frustration about never being able to find 'serious clients,' to (I'm ashamed to admit), anger and resentment toward those who I felt were wasting my time and efforts and deliberately trying to make me look bad. (Irrational, I know, yet it often felt that way at the time.)

Then I realised that the fitness and motivational industries had done a real number on both personal trainers and the clients they serve.

Trainers were told that if a client really and truly wants results, they'd do what's asked of them, no questions asked...and that, of course, if they didn't, that they were wasting both their own time and their trainers' because they simply weren't serious enough about getting results. At the same time, those who were trying to lose weight and get into shape were being made to feel that they were lazy, unmotivated and so stupid that they couldn't figure out that an apple was a better choice of snack than a chocolate bar.

In short, getting into great shape was becoming a lose-lose proposition for all concerned. And one that was adversarial in nature too. Trainers were fighting a battle against 'lazy' clients and clients were in combat with diets and exercise programs they hated, and that simply didn't work for them.

The trouble was, despite all this battling, no one was winning… and they couldn't.

So, against the backdrop of all this battling, I realised something that no one else seemed to be talking about. **The way we were approaching fitness and health simply was not working anymore…and perhaps it never did!**

The idea of eating less and moving more sounds so simple and obvious, yet so few people seemed able to pull this off in any way whatsoever, and those that did only managed it for a short period of time at best.

It struck me then that all of the motivational 'just do it… winners never quit and quitters never win… if you can conceive it and believe it you can achieve it' quotes in the world simply weren't working either. 'Just do it' sounded great, but what if 'doing it' is what you're struggling with most of all?

'Winners never quit' sounds cool too, but what if you've never seen yourself as a winner and have never experienced winning in the first place?

'Conceive, believe, achieve' sounds amazing, but what if you really DON'T believe?

No-one was asking these questions, let alone trying to answer them. Instead it seemed that we were simply insisting that accomplishment and achievement was as simple as living the quotes… even though so few seemed to be able to do so.

So I made it *my* business to find the answers. And I realised something pretty quickly…

Most of the failures, struggle, stresses and problems we face in pursuing our goals lie not in the goals themselves (pretty much any goal is achievable when you break it down into logical steps), but rather in the fact that we fail to do the one thing that is guaranteed to help us succeed in our quest to reach them. Trouble is, failing to do that one thing guarantees that we never will!

The one thing?

WE FORGET TO RELEASE THE BRAKES

Picture this…

You get into your car, start the engine, put your foot on the gas and… nothing. No movement at all, just the noise of the engine turning over.

Confused, you check that the car is in gear, hit the gas a little harder and hear the engine give a satisfying roar as the revs increase – yet once more, nothing. You're going nowhere.

Frustrated now, you floor the gas, the engine screams, the whole car vibrates and starts to roll forward just a little as bit by bit, the power of the engine overcomes the inertia of a ton of glass, metal and upholstery, yet because you're concerned about the noise coming from the engine, the smell of burning rubber coming from the wheels and the intense vibration coming from everywhere you decide to stop….to quit…you'll take your journey another day, you decide.

Just as you're about to switch off the engine and call your mechanic, you look down and experience a Homer Simpson 'Doh!' moment as you realise that you still had your parking brake in place. No wonder you weren't going anywhere!

You release the brake, lightly tap the gas and roll easily and quietly out of the driveway and set out for your destination… at last!

Why the story about cars and brakes?

Because it describes EXACTLY why most of your fitness and fatloss attempts fall flat on their face. In your effort to 'just do it', you're setting out on your journey without doing the most important thing you could possibly do to assure your success.

You're setting out without releasing the brakes!

— Starting a diet while you still have processed, high sugar, high carb food in your cupboards and refrigerator?

Brake!

If you own it you WILL eat it.

— Starting an exercise program without setting aside specific times to exercise?

Brake!

If you can't say EXACTLY when your training will take place, then you're unlikely to train at all. 'Today' or 'later' isn't the same as '6:15 am every day' for example.

— Setting out without a clear purpose and a deep and meaningful reason for pursuing them?

Brake!

A big enough 'why' will keep you on the straight and narrow when times get tough, yet a small one (or none at all) will guarantee you'll quit every time.

These are just 3 examples, yet they clearly show how most attempts at getting into great shape are lost before they even get started, as driving with the brakes on is simply too hard, too tiring, too boring and lack any real power to make anyone want to commit to doing the work required to get the results.

On the other hand, releasing the brakes makes it all very easy for the simple reason that all of your efforts can be used to move you forward – rather than having to fight against the pull of those things that are holding you back.

You 'get' this, right? But how do you actually implement releasing the brakes so that you can benefit from all the forward momentum you're going to gain?

Easy!

Simply identify the biggest 3-5 brakes in each of the following areas:

- **Time** – what time brakes are keeping you from doing what you need to do in order to get the results you want to get? Where is time being used poorly? Where is time being wasted? What could you do to get more time?

- **Inspiration** – what kind of things are present in your life that are sapping your motivation and inspiration? What 'motivation thieves' are currently making life harder for you than it could and should be?

- **Clarity** – what are you not clear about, need to learn more about or want more information about? Lack of clarity is a BIG brake!

- **Relationships** – what relationship brakes are present that are making it hard to focus on your goal? WHO is getting in the way of your progress?

- **Nutrition** – what nutrition brakes are in your way that are keeping you from achieving your goal? Too many carbs? Processed foods? Snacking?

- **Exercise** – What elements of your exercise program are acting like brakes? Exercises you don't like? Gym you hate? Program that takes too long?

Once you've identified at least 3 brakes in each area, identify WHY they are brakes and how they actually affect your ability to progress toward your goals.

For instance, a relationship brake may be that you feel guilty about leaving your family for an hour in the evening while you go to the gym, because they already see so little of you due to work commitments. An exercise brake may be that you can't stand cardio training because everyone tells you that you have to do it to get results, and because of this you don't end up training at all.

Identify why each brake IS a brake and how the brake actually stops you: "I feel guilty leaving the house again after getting home from work, so I stay home with the family instead, but end up doing nothing but sitting on the sofa, watching TV, eating…and getting fatter."

It's important that you tell the truth, the whole truth and nothing but the truth while answering these questions. After all, the truth will set you free…as you'll soon see!

Finally, come up with 3-5 solutions that allow you to release each brake in each area where you're stuck.

Feel guilty about coming home late then going back out again?

Could you get up earlier and hit the gym on the way to work? Could you buy some fitness equipment and train at home? Could you make it fun and engage your kids in your plans to get into great shape?

In all 3 examples above, there's a solution for releasing the brakes. Pick one, or better still, create your own.

Do this for all of the primary brakes before you even think of putting your foot 'on the gas' and getting going in pursuit of your goals.

I know what you're thinking. Sounds like a lot of work, right? Maybe, but so is failing. So is starting but never finishing. So is never ever seeing the results you so desperately want to see in return for all your efforts.

Yet the 30 minutes this exercise will take to complete can change your life. Just 30 minutes and the brakes will release and with less effort than ever before you'll be moving along in the direction of your goals.

Just 30 minutes.

Ask the questions. Answer the answers.

Release the brakes and no matter how big your goal, your success is guaranteed…you'll see!

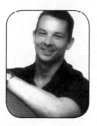

About Dax

Dax Moy is the guy you call when your dreams are too small.

A best-selling author with several titles related to self-development, personal growth, goal-achievement and holistic health as well as being a recognised member of The World Fitness Elite, Dax is a world- renowned expert in human performance – who is regularly sought out for his opinions on developing performance strategies that really work.

Dax has been seen on BBC News, ITV's *'This Morning'* Show, Ch4's 'You Are What You Eat', *CBS News and in The New York Times, The Washington Post, The Financial Times, The Evening Standard* and magazines such as *Men's Health, Men's Fitness, Health and Fitness, Glamour, Vogue* and *Cosmopolitan* among many others.

Dax is known as a coach who's dedicated to bringing out the greatness in others through his laser-focused ability to ask the questions that count, and finding the answers that inspire rapid and dramatic change in his clientele. His clientele includes Royalty, A-list celebrities, Actors, Musicians, Politicians and CEO's.

To learn more about Dax Moy –'The Guy You Call When Your Dreams are Too Small,' and to get a free copy of his special report *'The Biggest Lie - The TRUTH About Why Your Life Isn't Working Out'* visit: www.IAmDaxMoy.com

CHAPTER 3

FEMALE STRENGTH TRAINING: DO YOU WANT A LEANER, STRONGER, BETTER, BODY?

BY ANDREW "BO" TINAZA

I will admit that I personally enjoy resistance strength weight training and believe it is needed for optimal performance and physique goals for both males and females. I began experimenting with strength training in hopes of enhancing my athletic ability at the age of 13. And yes, like many teenage boys, I too began with the standard bicep curl. I attended a high school that had a successful powerlifting reputation for both girls and boys. The popularity of the powerlifting program at my high school resulted in a large number of teenagers within the school, especially the athletes, wanting to learn the "big lifts" such as barbell deadlift variations, barbell squat variations, bench press, and other Olympic lifts in their training programs.

The majority of the training programs that were designed for us and we participated in, may not have been the most organized programs, but they seemed to be showing results and getting the job done. If I had the knowledge back then that I have today, my high school strength training program would surely have been set up much differently. Although the programs were not complete training programs, I always included the "big lifts" which enhanced our athletic abilities, along with enhancing our physical appearance. You may be thinking, "of course you had good physiques! You were high school teenagers with accelerated metabolism, energy, activity levels and more." While this indeed may have played a part, not only teens have the ability to improve upon those fitness factors. You may or may not be correct. But everyone should understand that they have the ability to improve their metabolism, energy, and activity levels.

Following high school I completed my undergraduate degree in Kinesiology with the hopes of one day training college and professional athletes. After further consideration, I declined an offer to pursue a strength and performance coaching career at a Division I Collegiate program and rather decided to become an independent fitness trainer with the intent that taking this route would allow me to access and help a larger demographic of people needing fitness guidance. I wanted to work with all types of people that would include athletes, but not be limited to solely athletes. Fast-forward a quick three years and I now have a semi-private training facility in which the majority of the member base falls within the general population category. To say the least, I am so thankful to be able to wake up everyday and do what I am passionate about.

Helping people achieve their health and fitness goals and witnessing these changes which will enhance their lives in so many ways is simply amazing. One of the more popular programs at our facility is the small group strength training, which also happens to be one of my favorite sessions to coach. It may come as a surprise, but the strength program is very popular with many female members. These women work hard during their sessions, incorporating heavy deadlift variations, squat variations, press variations, chin ups, pull ups, calisthenics variations, along with other exercise options. These specific exercises are all geared to help gain lean muscle, improve metabolism, and empower the individual.

I see that today's women are becoming more comfortable and open to the idea of incorporating results-based driven strength and power program with their exercise routine as opposed to the past. Although the popularity has risen, I still have women coming into our facility and bringing up the many different myths associated with female strength-training. I could create a never-ending list that I have heard concerning strength-training for females, but I will discuss the five misconceptions that are brought to my attention on a regular basis.

#1. "I DON'T WANT TO BECOME 'BULKY' AND LOOK TOO MASCULINE FROM LIFTING WEIGHTS."

This is, without a doubt, the number one myth that I hear from females, questioning the results of strength training. First and foremost, women naturally have an uphill battle when it comes to becoming "she-hulk" due to their lower testosterone levels, the hormone mainly responsible for muscle gain, as compared to men. The average male has approximately 15 to 20 times the amount of testosterone as compared to the average female. A lot of males, myself included, struggle to reach their desired hypertrophy (muscle size increase) goals. This simple fact alone helps to explain that females with lower testosterone levels will have a difficult time gaining a lot of muscle hypertrophy.

Most females see female body builder pictures and instantly think that strength training is what causes those physiques. The majority of female body builders who have extreme muscle mass have a strict training program geared for those fitness goals, while some are genetically more able to gain muscle mass and others supplement with testosterone or steroids to reach those extreme muscle gains. Strength training will help to gain muscle but this isn't the culprit behind the "bulky" look for the general female population. Exercise, including strength training, may lead to individuals believing they can overeat or feel they need to eat more. This will cause an increase in body fat which will, in turn, result in the "bulky" look that females fear. Strength training will lead to increases in lean muscle, which will cause more calories to burn post workout and while at rest. This is perceived as improved metabolism. If a reasonable whole foods nutrition program is kept, fat loss, along with revealing lean muscle, will achieve the "toned" aesthetic that is sought after.

#2. "I NEED MORE 'CARDIO' SO I CAN GET THAT LEAN ATHLETIC LOOK."

The majority of people refer to "cardio" as steady state aerobic training such as jogging, elliptical, Stairmaster, and other steady state methods. I don't have any problem with these methods of training. I believe any type of physical activity will benefit an individual. Contrary to popular belief, steady state aerobic training is not the first training option for optimal fat loss. I believe any type of physical activity is a benefit and if you enjoy it, then, by all means, include it within your training schedule. The #1 training option for fat loss purposes is resistance (strength) training. This is because strength training causes your muscles to break down and rebuild over the next 24-48 hrs. The amount of energy and calories used during this process causes your metabolic rate to increase during this period of time. This process is known as excess post-exercise oxygen consumption, or, "the afterburn effect."

In short, strength training will boost your metabolism because more muscle is gained, which helps your body burn calories more efficiently and can result in more effective fat loss.Steady State Cardio for the most part only burns calories while you actually train and doesn't continue like a solid strength training session would.

#3. "STRENGTH TRAINING IS TOO DANGEROUS."

We will keep this one short because a lot of explanation isn't necessary. Anything can be dangerous under the wrong circumstances. Participating in sports, driving cars, riding a bike, walking down the street and so on can be "dangerous" if you are not properly prepared. If you take the time to learn the basic movements, or better yet, find someone who can teach the proper techniques and supervise, then safety is no longer an issue, and you can reap the benefits of including strength training in your exercise regime.

#4. "I DON'T WANT TO TRAIN LIKE A MAN."

I don't know where or when training became gender specific? A lot of females believe that only men should lift heavier weights and complete exercises such as deadlifts, squats, overhead presses, pull/chin ups, and other strength training methods. At my facility, both males and females have a strength-training component within their training program. Everyone completes the necessary movement patterns to enhance their overall fitness levels (squat, hinge, pull, push, single leg, lunge, core). This doesn't mean that everyone should do the same exact training program, but rather both men and women can greatly benefit from heavier resistance training. There isn't an exercise that is strictly for males or strictly for females.

#5. "LIFTING LIGHT HIGH REPS WILL GET ME A 'TONED' LOOK."

If you use a light weight for high repetitions you won't provide your body with a challenging enough stimulus that it must adapt to. You will just be moving and your body won't be challenged to make any type of serious changes. This is a basic principle of strength training, the principle of overload. In order to keep making gains, the exercise must become more difficult. Without this increase, our bodies adapt to the workload and eventually will plateau and even regress. I don't think people spend their time and energy to go to the gym and train without expecting to see results or changes.

While these myths may be common beliefs, they are easily disproven and overshadowed by the many benefits that a proper strength-training program can have for the female population. Here are some examples:

1. Helps control weight and preserve muscle mass: With increase in age comes decrease in muscle mass. What is one method to counteract this nonsense? If you guessed strength training, you are correct. If you don't preserve and enhance your muscle mass through strength training you are most likely going to have an increase in body fat. Who wants that?

2. Weight Control: A proper strength-training program will help to reduce body fat and burn calories more efficiently because muscle burns more calories than fat. This is a good reason to add some strength work.

3. Reduces the risk of osteoporosis: Strength training can help your bones grow stronger and maintain strength. Unfortunately women will naturally begin to lose bone density as they age, which will increase the chances of developing osteoporosis.

4. Helps prevent injury: When you gain muscle through strength training, you help protect your joints from injury and improve your balance and coordination. This help you in all facets of life, especially as we age.

5. Empowerment: The amount of confidence, independence, and improved self-esteem that a female can attain through strength training is endless. Each obstacle that she overcomes while at the gym will transfer over into her daily life. Suddenly, tasks such as lifting heavier objects, fitting into smaller jeans, happiness with her appearance, and simply being stronger and more confident are all effects that are lasting. Some other benefits include:

- Boosts Basal Metabolic Rate (BMR)
- Improves metabolism
- Lowers blood pressure
- Decreases risk of diabetes
- Improves posture and helps eliminate back and neck discomfort
- Stress reduction, mood improvement
- Helps increase mental alertness and energy levels
- Improves cardiovascular health
- Strengthens joints, ligaments, and tendons
- Releases endorphins

So what now? You may have already skipped down to this section to see what I would recommend.

First you must remember that a training program should be relative to each individual's fitness levels. I have females that I coach who can barbell deadlift 200 to 300+ lbs. with proper technique and form and some who may start with strictly bodyweight variations. Others may need to start with simple body weight exercises until they can progress to dumbbells, kettlebells, barbells, and so on. So don't go and attempt a 500 lb. deadlift just yet. If you are completely new to strength training, I would recommend searching for an expert in the field that can help you design a program for your specific needs.

Generally speaking, I believe everyone should incorporate and establish the basic movements within their strength-training program. These movements included squat, hinge, push, pull, single leg stance, lunge and core. Ideally, I would have the majority of females start on a 2 to 3 day per week full body strength training program with at least a day in between each strength session. We would work each movement to create a balanced program that will enhance all the muscle groups.

Here is an example outline of a full body training session that incorporates strength training:

- Foam roll, dynamic warm up/movement prep, core activation
- Power Training
- Strength Training
- Density/assistance supplement Training
- Energy System Training
- Post-Workout flexibility

The key is to incorporate all the necessary movements during your training session. We want to develop a balanced program that will get you results. We usually would set up the programs in a training program A and training program B format. For example, if you decide to train 3x per week you would complete training program "A" on Monday, "B" on Wednesday, and "A" again on Friday. The following week you would switch it around so that you complete "B" on Monday, "A" on

Wednesday, and "B" on Friday. It is important to also progressively overload or modify your training accordingly as you progress.

Sample Training Program "A"

Foam Roll, Dynamic warm up/movement prep:

1A. Plank Variation 2x 20-30 seconds

1B. Leg Raise 2 x 20-30 seconds

Minimal rest between each exercise and 30 sec. – 1 min. rests between each super set.

Power:

2A. Jumping Variation (Box Jumps, Squat Jumps, Broad Jump) 3 x 6

3A. Squat Variation (Body Weight, Goblet, Front, Back) 4 x 6-10

3B. Pull Variation (Horizontal-BW, DB, KB, BB) 4 x 6-10

Minimal rest between each exercise and 1 min. – 2 min. rest between each super set.

4A. Single Leg Movement (Split Squat, Lunge, Step Up, Side Lunge) 3 x 10-12

4B. Pull Variation (Vertical-BW, DB, KB, BB) 3x 10-12

4C. Push Variation (Horizontal-BW, DB, KB, BB) 3x 10-12

Minimal rest between each exercise and 1 min. – 2 min. rests between each super set.

Sample Training Program "B"

Foam Roll, Dynamic warm up/movement prep:

1A. Plank Variation 2x 20-30 seconds

1B. TRX Fall Out 2 x 20-30 seconds

Minimal rest between each exercise and 30 sec. – 1 min. rests between each super set.

2A. Swing Variation (KB, DB, Ball,) 2 x 8

2B: Jamball Slam 2 x 8

3A. Hinge Variation (Body Weight, Romanian Deadlift, Kettlebell Deadlift, Trap Bar Deadlift, Barbell Deadlift) 4 x 6-10

3B. Push Variation (Vertical-DB, KB, BB) 4 x 6-10

Minimal rest between each exercise and 1 min. – 2 min. rest between each super set.

4A. Single Leg Movement (Split Squat, Lunge, Step Up, Side Lunge) 3 x 10-12

4B. Pull Variation (Horizontal-BW, DB, KB, BB) 3x 10-12

4C. Push Variation (Vertical-BW, DB, KB, BB) 3x 10-12

Minimal rest between each exercise and 1 min. – 2 min. rest between each super set.

<u>Bonus:</u>

You can add some energy system training ("finisher") at the end of each session, and/or on the days you are not strength training, if you are at a proper fitness level.

High Intensity Interval Training (HIIT) is an effective training protocol especially for fat loss purposes.

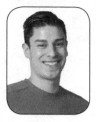

About Andrew ("Bo")

Andrew Tinaza, known by the nickname "Bo", is the owner of Fitness Ablaze Training Center located in Olympia, WA. His unique and effective training and coaching strategies have quickly established him as an elite fitness expert. He demonstrates a lot of passion for health and fitness, which has influenced many people throughout his area.

His methods include a mixture of power training, strength training, functional training and conditioning. Bo specializes in providing effective and efficient training to a large demographic of people ranging from younger child/teens to the general adult population to the elite athlete to the elderly. He believes everyone has the ability to improve their fitness levels and achieve their individual goals, which will only enhance the overall quality of their lives.

Bo received a degree in Kinesiology (Exercise Science) from Western Washington University. He currently is a Certified Personal Trainer (CPT) through the American Council on Exercise (ACE), Certified Strength and Conditioning Specialist (CSCS) through the National Strength and Conditioning Association (NSCA), *Training For Warriors* Certified and his gym, Fitness Ablaze Training Center is also currently a *Training For Warriors* Affiliate. He is a strong believer in continuing education and improvement.

Bo is constantly surrounding himself with other elite fitness professionals while attending many seminars, workshops, and other events to further enhance his craft. He believes as a fitness professional he should always strive to become better so he can have the ability to reach out to more people and help influence more people through health and fitness.

To learn more about Andrew "Bo" Tinaza, you can visit: www.fitnessablaze. com. You can also contact him directly through phone: (360) 529-3925 or email: fitnessablaze@gmail.com

CHAPTER 4

REVLINE'S TRAVEL FITNESS 101

BY COREY SOUSA

You work too hard at the gym year round to let your business trips throw you off course. My name is Corey Sousa and I own and operate Revline Fitness. I started Revline two years ago after the realization that many of my clients travelled extensively—and having a brick and mortar gym only just wouldn't suffice. I train all kinds of people from CEOs to Rappers, models and daycare owners. Revline is based on the principles that in today's world we are ever so connected and fitness must be adapted to this notion. At the time I wrote this chapter, I've had clients on six continents this year alone and it's only March.

Nonetheless, even with all the travel, long hours worked, and never-ending demands of today's society, there is still no excuse not to keep yourself fit and in shape. There are apps, YouTube, Skype, BBM, Whatsapp, SMS, and yes, even phone calls are still an option. With that being said, nothing beats face-to-face interaction. That's a fact and that won't change in the near future. If it does, I probably will be out of a job! Yes, I do travel with some of my clients for special projects. This ensures adherence to the program 100% – that they will be in shape when working with tight deadlines. For the rest of my clients that I train online, I set up Skype weekly or bi-weekly meetings to ensure they are keeping up with the training program that I have left with them.

First time I travelled with my clients

The first road trip I took with clients was from Montreal to Toronto for a music awards show. It was only for five days, but I quickly realized how much people could become distracted from their routines when they are in unfamiliar or semi-familiar environments. From strategic food choices to fast food, and early morning wake ups to early morning partying, it was the complete flip side. This firsthand experience made me realise how much my clients needed accountability for their actions when they're gone. I realised those snap shots I would receive of clients working out at the hotel gym, or running outside in Revline gear, were not exactly representative of their entire trip.

Traditionally, yes, we would all train in a gym with a trainer 3-4 times a week, all be eating organic and clean and be the healthiest population ever. But that's not necessarily the case. So I had to be creative and find a system that my clients would actually follow when they are on the road. I came up with five principles that all Revline clients follow when they leave for trips, be it vacation or business.

FIVE PRINCIPLES FOR TRAVEL FITNESS
– HOW TO STAY ON TRACK WHILE TRAVELING

1. Pack accordingly (clothes aren't all you need)

Your business trip is all planned, you have your itinerary ready and all you have left to do is pack and jump in the cab to the airport. One essential thing every person with a travel schedule should have at home is a fitness travel pack. This is a bag with several items that you don't touch unless you are throwing them in your suitcase. This is so that you are not chasing after any items that are missing in the basement from your work out in between commercials last weekend. This fitness kit is perfect for the light traveller in that it won't weigh you down if you only have a carry-on, and it won't take up space if you already have a lot of stuff. Here are the essentials in the fitness kit:

- Suspension Trainer

- Mini-Bands

- Travel Bands

- Note Pad
- Timer
- Gliders

This is not a heavy investment by any stretch and with all these items, throw in a few calisthenics and you can do a total body workout in your hotel room. All of these items are easy to travel with and are relatively inexpensive. Each one of these items serves one essential purpose among others.

The suspension trainer is best served for effective posterior chain exercises. My favorite is the inverted row and with the door adaptor that it comes with makes it perfect for any hotel room. Mini bands are great for activating your glutes and hip muscles. After a long period of time sitting in cabs, airports, planes, it's always a good idea to fire up the glutes and avoid gluteal amnesia. Make sure to get your rest first after the long flight before performing these exercises as this is the best form of recovery.

Travel bands are great for any of your push exercises, just tie them to the doorknob and you can do your punches and chest flys. You can leave them free standing and do your shoulder exercises as well. Gliders are great for reverse lunges, side lunges, glute and ham bridges. Any exercises lower body dominant are a plus. You can throw in a travel band for resistance or as is.

It's important to note that when training in your hotel room with limited resistance, mass gains will not be a priority. With that being said, you can still get an effective workout for endurance and/or cardio by designing it accordingly. This is where the timer comes into play. A timer is probably the most essential item, as now being on the road you may not be able to squeeze in a full hour workout, so you'll be forced to combine exercises – the most efficient way to train high volume or HIIT (high intensity interval training). You will keep an elevated heart rate, and lactic acid build up will lead to an increase in production of Growth Hormone and therefore an increase in fat loss.

2. Plan accordingly

The second principle is to plan accordingly. Basically, know your surroundings of where you are going. Take the time sometime before you leave or have someone do it for you to check it out. Scout the surrounding area of your hotel so you find out where the closest grocery store is located. Take note of the restaurants in the surrounding area because if something comes up (things always come up) then you can at least have a backup plan for where to eat and it will be reasonably healthy.

I can't stress this enough, but throw some fruit in your bag and eat it at the airport, whether or not it is a banana (yes, I know banana's contain a lot of sugar), at least that can tide you over until you reach your destination (assuming you've eaten properly throughout the day). There's nothing worse than being on the plane and having to eat plane food, not to mention how pricey it can get.

3. Be accountable for your actions

This one is simple in theory – have someone other than you be accountable while you travel. Write down what you are eating and keep a food and exercise log with you, It's easy to skew them in your favor and think you 'ate healthy' when you don't write them out. When you write down that extra donut or the few beers and it is written down, then the calories (or macros) that come with it cannot be disputed. In your itinerary for the trip, schedule in your workouts while you will be gone. At the end of the trip, reflect and write out if you worked out. Yes or No? And why or why not? What will have to change the next time for improved efficiency? Evaluate and make appropriate changes for the next trip.

If you're feeling confident this can be done with ease, you can take it a step further and have the macro break down of the foods you ate. There are great apps that do most of the work for you. Again, it's about seeing the results in front of you. Most people think they eat healthier than they actually are eating. I make every Revline client I work with fill out a 48-hour log from our assessment day to the next time we train, so they can be held accountable.

Always tell your trainer when you are out of town. Ideally, he will be the other person holding you accountable. Have a Skype session with him or have him call/email/Facebook/tweet you while you are away so that you can be held accountable. You should feel comfortable enough with your trainer to ask for this kind of accountability. If you are not, this may indicate a problem on various levels – but that's another chapter. Just ask a friend, don't ask your mom, she'll always justify for you why you didn't adhere to the plan in your favor!

4. Stay Hydrated (coffee doesn't count)

Most of us know the importance of water and it is essential for life. Unfortunately, most people don't realise they are not drinking the daily required amount of water. If you add the fact that people are out of their normal environment and have a packed schedule because they are travelling, water intake declines even more than usual. Water intake should be 30-40 mL for every kilogram you weigh, that translates to 2-4L if you weigh between 110 and 220 lbs. – the average male or female falls within this weight category. It's safe to say that roughly ¼ of your water intake comes from food and the rest will be drinkable water. If you drink a lot of coffee (like I do), which actually dehydrates you, then add a 1 to 1 ratio of coffee to water in addition to what you normally should be drinking.

Thirst is an indicator that you are beginning to be dehydrated, however, it is not the first sign. While this is a good indicator that your body needs water, at this point 1-2% of your total body weight has already been lost due to dehydration, so don't wait! Also, the biggest part of why we should drinking more water is that our lack of water intake can be misinterpreted by our minds into thinking we are hungry. Sometimes that hungry feeling is actually our bodies telling us that we need more water, so drink more water and avoid those hunger feelings, because if you're like me, being hungry means being in a bad mood!

5. Create a new habit while you are on the road and make sure to stick with it when you get back

This one is easy to start but hard to follow. What I mean by that is it is easy to start a new habit when you are in a different environment. Everything is new to you, so you can take the time to set your day up as you wish. You also have less distractions; chances are your family isn't with you, neither are all of your co-workers, therefore you can spend more time doing what you want to do. The problem then becomes keeping this habit when you return to your normal environment (i.e., home). Everything was just as it was before you left, so you immediately tend to your natural tendencies.

Creating a habit generally takes three weeks. Knowing this, the best way to position yourself so that your habit will succeed even after you return from your trip is to look at exactly how many days you are gone. If you are gone for only a week, start your habit one week prior to the trip and then make sure it lasts one week after you get home. If you are gone for two weeks, try to keep the momentum going after you get home. You can play with how you work out in the three weeks, and of course, everyone is different and can take longer or shorter depending on the type of person you are. Here are four habits that I typically suggest to clients on the road to make travel easier:

1) Sleep more – improve cognitive function and proper rest for your muscles

2) Schedule your meals – reduce cortisol levels (stress) and hunger pains (ghrelin)

3) Train at the same time every day on your trip

4) Time is something many people wish they had more of: so be more productive – watch less television, go to sleep 15 minutes earlier, wake up an hour earlier

Implementing any and all of these will increase your fitness level, mental capacity and give you a better quality of life. At first, it definitely will take getting used to doing. Like anything else we do, we have to do it until it becomes mindless. If you start to taper off, reflect on when you first started the new habit and reflect on the benefits of it and it will help you return to the habit.

Example workout – Total Body Workout (21 Minutes)

Exercise	Reps/Time
Band Walks (length of room and back)	—
Inverted Rows	30 seconds
Shoulder Flys (w/bands)	30 seconds
Push ups (use bed for females)	30 seconds
Core Get Ups	30 seconds
Rest for 1 min -	**Repeat sequence 3x**
Goblet Squats (or Jump Squats)	30 seconds
Band Pull Aparts	30 seconds
Reverse Lunges (use Gliders)	30 seconds
Shoulder T's or Y's off bed	30 seconds
Hip Bridges	30 seconds
Rest for 1 min -	**Repeat sequence 3x**

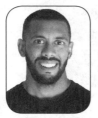

About Corey

Corey Sousa is founder of Revline Fitness, a leading fitness company in Montreal, Canada. Extensive travel is part of everyday life when dealing with CEOs/musicians/artists/actors who cannot commit to one gym in one city, and Corey has created a personalized program to help even the most frequent flier.

Corey also provides gym management and training services remotely to his Los Angeles and Toronto clients. Being away from Montreal, he needed a solution for his current clients. Today there are Revline trainers in multiple cities that are all connected through Revline and their online systems.

Corey has spent his time learning from the masters in the Training and Sports industry. Having played a variety of team sports throughout high school, he then turned his attention to training at the age of 16. He has had the privilege of training along many professional athletes from the NHL, UFC, MLB, MLS, NFL, and MLB among others.

Corey's training methods include Olympic weightlifting, functional training, calisthenics, as well as many other methods to produce optimal strength and performance gains. His specialty is adaptability to his clientele – who travel extensively – and consistently monitoring their nutrition for optimal results.

Corey has been coached and mentored by some of the top fitness coaches and professionals in the world. He attends seminars nationally and internationally and continually studies everything he can – from fitness to nutrition to psychology. He takes a holistic approach to training and tries to get the most out of the 168 hours in a week from his clients.

For more information call:
(514) 518 - 0750 or
(310) 923 - 6882

Or visit:
www.revlinefitness.com

CHAPTER 5

REVIVING YOUR METABOLISM

BY WILL CLEWIS

One morning while sitting at my desk in the gym office, my phone rings. I answer AMP Fitness, this is Will, and on the other end of the phone was a woman who was in desperate need. She explained, her whole life she's been an athlete. There was never a time that she remembered having to go on a strict diet. She was a former 100-meter sprinter in college and so she's always been naturally lean and in great health. Once college was over, things began to take a turn for the worse. She was no longer physically active, now she was working full time, and even worse, her health had took a turn for the worse. Reminiscing she cried, I'm so ashamed that I have let myself go like this. I'm 50 pounds heavier, my metabolism is dead and I just don't know what to do. In great desperation she asked, "Could you help me Will?" I said, "Of course! Come in and I will show you exactly how we can fix your broken metabolism."

Many people believe if you're skinny you have a high metabolism, and if you are obese, your metabolism is slow. This is not always the case. So before we can get into reviving your metabolism, you must first understand exactly what it is.

Metabolism is the whole range of biochemical processes that occur within humans (or any living organism) to maintain life. These biochemical processes allow us to grow, reproduce, repair damaged tissues, and respond to our ever-changing environment. Think of metabolism as the harmonizer of two bodily functions that are the opposite of each other. These bodily functions are catabolism and anabolism.

Catabolism is the process of the body breaking down food we ingest and converting it into fuel or energy for the many functions our bodies do. Everything from blinking, thinking, moving, all the way to transporting blood requires energy. Anabolism creates bigger things out of small things and uses up energy in the process. It allows the body to create new cells and maintain all the tissues. The body uses simple molecules to create complex ones. In the same way a builder will use simple building blocks, such as bricks, to create a house. Anabolic reactions in our bodies utilize a few simple chemicals and molecules to manufacture a myriad of finished products. An increase in muscle mass, or a scab forming around a wound would be examples of anabolism. Your body does this constantly all day and night— Determining whether we should breakdown cells (catabolism) or build new cells (anabolism).

So now we have an idea of exactly what metabolism is now we can investigate how it slows down.

I'm going to share with you four ways that cause your metabolism to take a dip. They are diet, hormone dysfunction, sleep deprivation, and exercise. Regulating these things are critical in making sure your metabolism is running at optimal performance.

1. First we will begin with SAD (standard American diet). Most Americans have a diet that is high in refined sugars and starches. Just think about the typical breakfast foods people indulge in. You have donuts, cereal, breakfast bars, smoothies, etc., and these foods are jam-packed with sugars. Now the one thing our bodies hate more than anything is elevated blood sugars. It literally can't stand it. Over extended periods of time of shoveling sugars into your body, and continuing to spike your insulin, a process calls insulin resistance occurs. Let me walk you through it so you know exactly what happens inside your

body. Whenever you eat carbohydrates, your body converts them into glucose (sugar). Once your brain has sensed a spike in your blood sugar, it sends a signal over to your pancreas to release a hormone called insulin. Insulin is the transporter that delivers this glucose to your Liver and Muscles. Think of it as the hormone that gives life to the cells.

2. When you have more of a hormone in the body than what you should, the cells have to protect themselves from these hormones because they are so powerful. The only way insulin can open the door to this cell is through something called a receptor. Think of it like a lock and key. Insulin comes in and plugs in to the receptors then pumps in sugar, protein, fat, vitamins and minerals into the cells. When insulin resistance develops, the cells look at insulin as being toxic. So what happens is the cells pull those receptors inside, so insulin can no longer get in. When your body can't remove sugar via insulin, the sugar has to be dealt with. Remember your body hates this state more than anything. So what happens is your body converts it to triglycerides and stores it as fat. When you over-secrete insulin for so long that your cells now view it as toxic, it won't let any sugars in. This is another term for type two diabetes.

3. The next reason your metabolism slows down is because of sleep deprivation. Recent studies have shown that Americans are only getting on average about five hours of sleep. Two of the main reasons are stress, and not creating an environment conducive for rest. Picture this for a second. There is a mother in the kitchen washing dishes and her son is outside playing with a ball in the yard. His ball rolls underneath the car, which is sitting on blocks. The kid goes underneath the car to fetch the ball and the car falls. The mom sprints out the door, raises up the car and pulls her son from underneath. Now what just happened was she had a huge surge of cortisol and adrenaline released in her body. These are powerful hormones that are secreted in stressful situations. It's no different then you being yelled at by your boss at work. Now sleep is critical to our bodies. Think of

it as the workshop where you get all your energy, and fuel to prepare you to meet the demands of the next day. It's going to be virtually impossible to get a good nights rest when you have an influx of cortisol in your body.

4. Now the final way your metabolism comes to a screeching halt is through living a sedentary lifestyle. Statistically, obesity is at an all-time high. It has surpassed tobacco smoke as the number one cause of mortality in Americans. This is extremely saddening, because it is 100 percent controllable. Technology is so advanced now it has replaced the desire for people to get out and move. It is rare to see kids outside running around, playing basketball, roller blading, etc. Those activities have been replaced with video games, and digital activities. The lack of exercise, specifically strength training, will cause a decrease in muscle mass, which ultimately will cause you to burn less fat. The less muscle on your body, the lower your metabolic rate.

So now that we have learned a few things that cause your metabolism to slow down, lets look at what we need to do to revive it.

The most important thing is fueling your body with the proper nutrition. Studies have shown that frequent feedings approximately four to six times a day has been linked to increased metabolism. Your diet should include the following things: Proteins, Vegetables, Nuts and Seeds, some Fruit, a little starch, and no added sugars. We need protein for the building and repairing of tissue in our body. Protein-rich foods also include essential minerals, such as iron, magnesium, zinc, as well as B vitamins. Proteins should make up about 30% of our nutritional intake. Good sources of protein include chicken, fish, turkey, lean beef, pork, shellfish, and any gamey meat you like. Veggies and fruit are known to contain high amounts of vitamins, minerals, and fiber. These nutrients are vital for your body to function at optimum performance. Studies have proven that a diet high in fruits and veggies can protect against heart disease, cancer, and type two diabetes. These good sources of carbohydrates should make up about 40% of your nutritional intake. These are lower on the glycemic index and won't spike up your insulin levels as much as carbohydrates loaded with refined sugars. Aim for good quality fats daily. These fats should come from almonds, cashews, olive oil, flax seed, avocado, and lots of fish. A diet containing good fats has been shown to lower inflammation under the skin, and promotes a healthy functioning heart. These fats should count as 30% of your dietary intake.

Next we have to keep your hormones happy and functioning at a high capacity. Now earlier in the chapter we talked about constantly shoving sugars in the body causes insulin spikes, and insulin spikes chronically would lead to insulin resistance and fat gain. So what we need to do to avoid this is to limit the amount of refined sugars we consume. The only time these sugars should be consumed is after weight-bearing exercise. During this time your body will be primed and prepped to best handle these sugars. Instead of storing these sugars as fat, they will be absorbed by the muscle to help them recover from the exercise you just performed.

Furthermore to promote a healthy functioning metabolism we have to get restful nights sleep. First we should do an internal audit of our lives. Look and see what is causing you stress. I guarantee there are things that are serving you no purpose which you could stop now, and doing so would decrease your stress load which in turn will decrease your cortisol levels. The next step is to create what I call a sleep cave. It will require you to put away the cell phone, turn off the television, and any other light source in the room. These lights and blue screens will keep the brain active not allowing you to fully relax into a rested state. The next thing you'll need is to create some white noise, and make sure the temp in the room is appropriate. An easy way to kill two birds with one stone here is to turn on a fan. Studies have been linked to having a cooler room temp, and white noise equates to more restful sleep. Implement these today and watch your sleep patterns improve dramatically.

The final thing you'll need to incorporate into your daily life to maintain a high metabolism is exercise. This is non-negotiable. Exercise can be separated into two broad categories. You have Aerobics and Anaerobic. It's best to have a balance of all of these in order to get the most benefits from your exercise program. The goal of aerobic exercise is to improve the body's consumption of oxygen. Most common aerobic exercises are done at low to moderate levels of intensity, for longer periods of time. They begin with a warm up, exercises for about 20 to 25 minutes, and then finish off with a cool down. An example of aerobics would be going for a 20 minute run.

The next form of exercise is anaerobic. The goal of anaerobics is to increase strength, power, and muscle. During anaerobic training muscles are exercised at high levels of intensity for short spurts of time. This typically means no longer than two minutes. *Anaerobic* simply means *without air.* It allows our body to move with quick bursts of speed. Think of it as short, fast and intense training. Examples of this are sprinting, interval training, weight training, and plyometric training. This form of training is great for building muscle mass on the body which in turn is going to increase your metabolic rate or rate at which your body burns fat at rest. Thus increasing your metabolism.

To get the most benefit from your exercise program you should include a balanced dose of both of these forms of training. I highly recommend a 4-day training split. This means Monday/Wednesday you'll perform anaerobic exercise weight lifting at high intensity, and Tuesday/Thursday you'll perform aerobic exercise or like going for a run or hopping on a rowing machine for 20-25 minutes. Friday you'll rest and let your muscles recover, then Saturday jump back into some weight training.

So now after reading this chapter you understand the causes of a slowing metabolism. They are bad nutrition, hormone dysfunction, sleep deprivation, and living a sedentary lifestyle (lack of exercise). If you are struggling with any of these issues, and you've been having trouble losing weight, don't fret. Just follow the steps I laid out for you above and you'll be on your way to a faster, more efficient metabolism!

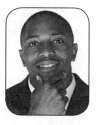

About Will

Will Clewis is an alumnus of The University of Central Oklahoma graduating in 2009 with a Bachelor's Degree in Education. Will received countless awards during his stint at the U of CO. He was named Six Time All American Line Backer, Defensive Player of the Year and Line Backer of the Year in 2006 and again in 2007. Will had aspirations of going to the NFL but decided to pursue his dream of Education and Fitness.

In 2009, Will moved to the Dallas-Fort Worth area and began his career as a 7th Grade History Teacher and Football Coach at Boles Junior High. After a few years of enlightening children and enhancing their physical abilities, he knew there was more. There was more to his gift and passion for fitness. In October 2010, Will founded AMP FITNESS LLC, which made its official debut in March 2011.

The DFW area had no clue what was about to happen next. AMP started off at a local park (Stovall Park) with 5 members. In November 2011, to accommodate its growth AMP moved to Deaver Park in Arlington, TX. By this time the word really began to spread about AMP Fitness. Throughout 2012, Will focused on providing top notch training and perfecting his business model with the dream of someday moving into his very own training facility. After countless hours of training clients (all the while still teaching), marketing, cleaning, training, marketing, training...did we mention marketing, in December 2012, Will hosted the Grand Opening of AMP Fitness on Kaltenbrun St. in Fort Worth, TX. This 2,000 sq.ft. tin building was truly a dream come true for him and his 50 members.

Throughout 2013, AMP's membership grew by leaps and bounds. By August 2013, AMP Kaltenbrun would see 100 consistent members on a day-to-day basis. He then realized it was time to step out on faith and focus on AMP full time. Will resigned from his teaching position in August 2013. In April 2014 Will announced to his almost 200 member gym they would be moving to a 5,000 sq.ft. state-of-the-art facility. Will and the AMP Fitness Family currently are located at the Berry St. location. This continued growth is a direct result of Will's desire to have AMP be a place where Men and Women come to simply "Reinvent" themselves. His customized program assists individuals in releasing the brakes off their internal and external lives. This, in turn, allows them to become the "BEST VERSION" of themselves also known as "Getting Better Everyday!"

Will is a certified trainer holding the American Muscle and Fitness Certification, Crossfit Level 1 Certification and Under Armour 360 Certification.

Will has also been recognized for his volunteer efforts throughout Fort Worth and the surrounding cities. Will has raised and donated thousands of dollars by hosting charity boot camps for Susan G. Komen Breast Cancer Awareness, Autism Speaks, Children's Cause for Cancer Advocacy (CCCA), The Wounded Warrior Project and many more.

In his leisure time, Will's hobbies include fishing, golfing, reading, grilling and spending time with family. Will is married to his beautiful wife Danielle, and has 3 children.

To learn more about AMP Fitness you can visit: www.ampfitnesstx.com

CHAPTER 6

THE FIVE BEST EXERCISES TO ADD MUSCLE AND SPEED UP YOUR METABOLISM

BY JOE BRAMMER

Hi! My name is Joe Brammer. If you are reading this book I imagine you would like to Seriously Transform your body for life, and do it in a sustainable way. I'm sure a lot of you have gone on diets and joined workout programs before but you did not stick with them because they were not sustainable.

In my opinion, the best way to transform your body long term is to speed up your metabolism. So what I want to talk to you about is the Five Best Ways to Build Muscle and speed up your metabolism – but first, I want to tell you a little about myself.

I grew up a pretty active kid in Des Moines, Iowa and was pretty thin, but in the 4th Grade we got a Super Nintendo and I spent a lot of time on the couch eating Cheetos and drinking Sunny Delight, while I battled my friends in Street Fighter 2…. A lot… of time… and as a result I put on a lot of weight. I was up to about 5 ft. 5 in. and 200 lbs. in the 6th grade.

In about 7th grade, I realized my weight had gotten out of control and I needed to do something about it. I think that realization had something to do with a combination of becoming interested in girls and being made fun of for being the fat kid. Both can be strong motivators, but honestly, being teased about being overweight was a very painful and real experience. The pain of being called fat and feeling like an outcast really pushed me to learn all that I could about losing weight and becoming physically fit.

So I took massive action. I ran and worked out out everyday and read and studied all that I could about weight loss and working out. By freshman year in High School, I was down to 135lbs! I had lost 65 lbs! After that I decided I wanted to get buff, so I started lifting weights every day religiously for about 4 years.

I started boxing and wrestling in high school, but in my senior year I was introduced to Brazilian Jujitsu, and from the first time I tried it, I was obsessed. As soon as high school was over, I began lifting weights and doing Brazilian jujitsu and Muay Thai every day, for 3 to 6 hours a day. After training for a few years and taking some amateur MMA fights, I decided I was going to go pro.

I moved out to Seattle, Washington to train with UFC Veteran Ivan Salaverry and Maurice Smith. After a few years, I was a Champion in Multiple organizations – fighting and beating some heavy competition like UFC star Michael Johnson. Well soon the UFC gave me a call, and I signed a contract with the biggest, baddest, fighting organization in the world, the UFC!

But even as a pro UFC fighter, I always kept studying the human body and all the different training programs, diet and nutrition programs and exercises out there. Not only did I read about them, but also I tried them – some worked and some did not, but I experimented. I had some of the best coaches and trainers in the world, and have worked with some of the top athletes in the sport and learned even more working with them.

But now I am retired, and instead of spending my time beating people down, I spend my time building people up. I own a body transformation center, Elite Edge Gym in Waukee, IA. I see hundreds of clients every day that do not have a lot of time, usually 30 to 40 minutes is all they have. So we have to make sure what we are doing is the most effective program in the shortest time possible with the least risk of injury.

You probably have a very busy schedule like most of our clients, and would like to maximize your time in the gym. When I first start working with a client who wants to lose weight and get more toned, we want to do it quicker and easier, we work to first increase their metabolism.

Metabolic rate is simply the rate at which we burn calories. If you consume 2000 calories a day and burn 2000 calories you will remain at the same weight.

My favorite way to increase metabolism is by increasing the amount of muscle on your body. Every pound of muscle on your body will require about 50 calories a day. One study found that base metabolic rate is boosted about 15% with regular weight training. Muscle is metabolically active and burns more calories than any other tissue.

To speed up your metabolism as much as possible, we want to add as much muscle as possible, so I want to give you the 5 Best Exercises for building more muscle. Focus on these exercises to speed up your fat loss and you will spend less time in the gym and more time with your friends and family.

#1 – THE SQUAT

This exercise is a must. It works all the muscles in your legs and is the first muscle-building exercise in our arsenal. Start off light and focus on your technique to begin with. Arch your back from the beginning to end of the movement. Stick your chest out and place your feet slightly wider than shoulder width apart. Start the movement by hinging your hips back; imagine someone has a rope around your waist and they pull it back slowly as you sit back, controlling your weight, like you are sitting in a chair. Your head needs to be back, and you look straight ahead.

I recommend for people just starting out with this movement to get a chair or a plyo box to sit down on. Go all the way down where the crease of the hip is just below the knee.

#2 – DEADLIFT

This is a great exercise for working almost all the muscles in your body and will build overall strength and add nice lean muscle to your backside. Start with a narrow stance and the bar about 6 inches in front of you on the floor. Reach down and grab the bar with your hands outside of your knees with a double overhand grip. Drop your hips down below your shoulders and roll the bar back and against your shins. Drive your heels into the mat and pull straight up keeping the weight on your heels tell you are standing upright. Squeeze your glutes and core at the top of the movement and do not hyper-extend your back. Lower the weight straight down by dropping your hips back and keeping the bar close to you.

#3 – HIP THRUST

This is one of my favorite exercises because it is the best movement to activate the glutes and is very, very simple to learn and very effective! Plus, who doesn't want a better butt? To do this move, place your shoulders on a flat bench and your feet flat on the floor. Have a partner help you lower a barbell right onto the crease of your hips. I recommend you get a barbell pad or wrap a towel around the bar, without the extra padding this can be uncomfortable. Once you have the bar in place simply thrust your hips straight up and extend towards the ceiling. Be sure to keep your heels in the mat and squeeze your glutes at the top of the movement.

#4 – BENCH PRESS

You have probably heard of this exercise before and for good reason. The bench press, when done properly, is the cornerstone of building a more defined and sculpted upper body. Here are a few tips to make this exercise safe and more effective. Lay on the bench and grab the weight barbell slightly wider than shoulder width apart. Slowly lower the weight down to your chest and gently touch, keep your butt on the bench and push up with a slight angle toward your head. End the movement with the bar over your mouth.

#5 – MILITARY PRESS

This is the best exercise to build up your shoulders and get that hourglass shape or V-shape up top. You can do this exercise with the weight in front or behind your head. Some people are less flexible and putting the barbell behind their head is very uncomfortable. You can do either variation. Make sure your shoulders are warmed up before you start.

Start with your feet slightly wider than shoulder-width apart. Either use a rack or clean the barbell up to your chest. Start with a weight you can handle with control and place hands a little wider than shoulder width. Slowly press the barbell overhead and make sure to keep your core tight by squeezing your core and glutes. Do not jerk the weight or use momentum, keep your shoulders back and lower the weight under control. If you cannot lower the weight slowly you need to go lighter until you can control the weight.

The name of this book is Rapid Body Makeover, so I want to give you guys all something you can use right away to transform your body. Here is a 6-week jumpstart program you can do with these five Exercises.

Warm-up – Do 8 of each with just bodyweight:

- Squat
- Alternating Lunges
- Pushup
- Fire Hydrants
- Lateral Lunge
- High knee

Day 1

    a. Squat 5 x 5

    b. Assisted Pullups – 2 x 4-6

    c. Bench Press 5x 5

    d. Hip Thrust 2 x10

    e. Romanian Deadlift 3 x 8

    f. Assisted/Pushups – 3 x 10

    g. Crunches on Physio ball 3 x12

Day 2 – Rest.

Day 3

    a. Deadlift 5x5

    b. Single Arm Dumbbell Row 3x8 ea. side

    c. Sumo Stance bodyweight Squat 2x10

    d. Military Press 4x8

    e. Reveres lunge 2x10

    f.   Squat Hold 3 x 20 sec

    g. Standing dumbbell wood chop 2 x 10 ea. side

Day 4 – Rest.

Day 5

    a. Barbell Bent Over Row – 2 x 5

    b. Single leg curls 2 x 10 ea.

    c. Farmers Walk 2 x 40 yards (hold dumbbells at sides and walk around)

d. Hip Thrust with hold at top for 3 sec 3 x 5

e. Renegade Row 3 x 8 ea. side

f. Abs Wheel 2 x 8

g. Plank 3 x 30 sec

Day 6 – Rest.

Day 7 – Rest.

Repeat this program for 6 weeks. If you have never done these exercises before, please work with someone who has experience and can help you with form. I would hate for you to get hurt before you have a chance to transform your body.

Ease into these exercises, please do not try to go all out the first day, especially on deadlifts or squats, get used to the movements and focus on getting your form correct. Review this chapter and the descriptions of each exercise before lifting to get the movements fresh in your mind.

You will be very sore, so make sure to stretch after you work out, drink at least a gallon of water every day and sleep 8 hours. This is very important, as you have to let your body recover; these lifts make you very sore because they incorporate so much muscle recruitment, which is why they speed up your metabolism so much. So to get maximum benefit and make your body transformation, you need to take recovery time serious.

So those are my **five best exercises** to get your metabolism stoked and those calories burning. Please feel free to contact me at: joe@eliteedgegym.com I would love to hear from you.

BONUS TIP: What is the most important meal of the day? I bet like 99% of people said breakfast. That really is not true though, the most important meal of the day is whatever you eat right after your workout!

After a hard workout, your body needs nutrients to repair and rebuild all the damage from the weight training session. Recovery is the most important aspect of training. If you are not recovered properly from a training session, your next workout session will suffer and your progress will stop.

There has been a lot of research from a lot of credible sources on what amount of protein to carbs ratio you should consume, and how soon after a workout. A lot of the research varies slightly, but they all agree you should have 10 to 30 grams of protein and 10 to 30 grams of carbs within 30 to 90 minutes after your workout.

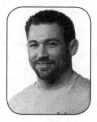

About Joe

Joe Brammer is Head Coach and founder of Elite Edge Gym. A fat loss expert who uses science-based training, targeted nutrition and mindset training to change peoples lives and create more pride, joy and passion in the lives of his clients. He is also a Certified Personal Trainer, former UFC Fighter, Certified Group Fitness Instructor, and the CEO of Elite Edge Gym.

Joe Brammer helps his clients Transform their lives through health and fitness.

Becoming an athlete and then a professional athlete, Joe has a passion for training and healthy living. He naturally gravitated toward the health and fitness world after his MMA career.

Joe's philosophy is you don't work out to lift more weights or lose weight, you work out to improve the quality of your life and get more joy and excitement out of every day.

You can connect with Joe at:
Joe@EliteEdgeGym.com

CHAPTER 7

A PILATES HOLISTIC APPROACH TO WELL BEING

BY TATTIANA GANDOLFO

Pilates healed and changed my body, my life and my purpose. By the age of 21, I had been an avid athlete playing soccer, a figure skater, dancer, practicing yoga, weight training, and a fashion and fitness model. A back and hip injury stopped me from doing what I loved which was to be active.

I was in the type of pain I would hear many people talk about. Lower back pain and Sciatica was something I had never experienced before. I had to find relief and I did not want to take any medicines my doctors were prescribing with bed rest. I needed to find a solution and to not mask my problem or wait for it to get worse. I started physical therapy to help me on my road back to recovery. There, in my therapist's office, was my cure. It was the answer to my lifelong search of how stay physically well inside and out. It was an exercise system based on physical and mental conditioning called Pilates.

My father, who passed away in 2004 from an aggressive Brain Tumor, believed in attaining perfect form, and started me at 14 years old with a personal trainer twice a week until I was 18. To be an athlete, he knew that I needed to have discipline, good body awareness, coordination, muscle strength and flexibility. He wanted me to learn how to care for my body and not to injure it when I entered the gym by either taking a group exercise class, training on the weight machines and using the free weights. As I went to gym with my father, he realized as I entered high school that I knew nothing about proper biomechanics and exercise safety. He was my role model, as I followed him around the gym from the treadmill, weight machines and stretching. I tried my hardest to replicate his exercises and movements after watching him complete his sets. My father would give me positive feedback to boost my confidence in a firm voice that resembled Arnold Schwarzenegger's. It was his strong Romanian accent and he was always someone you never messed with on the soccer field if the referees made a call, or if we were not performing at our best. One of my father's goals was to teach me how to work out without hurting myself, what muscles I should be feeling and especially improving my posture. He believed learning the right way at an early age would condition me to be injury-free and know what is and feels right from wrong.

Being a naïve teenager, I thought that I did know it all. After all, I studied the exercises, how to perform them, what muscle groups to work, what machines to use and at what weights, how to challenge my body with exercise choice and safety. As I laid down on my physical therapist's table, I was amazed but confused. It took an injury for me to find the perfect exercise system that taught me all of this in a few sessions. After the many years of being trained at the gym, a dancer since age 4, and as an athlete, I had never heard of this exercise method called Pilates. First, I found these Pilates exercises utilizing muscles that I never thought I had or knew how to engage. Second my "powerhouse" and shoulder, pelvis and back had to stabilize and integrate with exercises that required controlled movement and breathing. Third, I was hooked, healed and intrigued.

I wanted to learn everything there was about Pilates—especially how to help others—since it healed me and helped my body and mind fully recover. When you are in that sort of pain, your mind and emotions do not allow you to heal, your body is rigid and you worry way too much about if you will ever feel better. Most of us have felt that way before or have had seen loved ones deal with pain, whether it was a back condition, injury or some other form of pain. I needed to share this wealth of knowledge with others, and in 2001, I decided that this was my calling after considering a career in Art education. I wanted to teach Pilates. I wanted to touch the lives of others who I know would benefit as much as I did from such simple yet challenging exercises that integrated my entire mind, body and spirit. It was my calling.

Now 14 years later, I am still doing just that. I am helping others attain what physical well-being should feel like. It is without medicine, loud music or competition. Many of my clients who come in are stressed, slumped over, in pain, need to improve their sport or wellbeing. After working with hundreds of bodies, I am improving their everyday life by setting a strong foundation of optimum movement mechanics that help maintain the body position and alignment. It is a foundation that I call the ground floor. It is where the work starts, climbs up and reaches the skies limits. Without proper knowledge, skills or attention to detail, how do we climb upwards without starting from the ground floor of anything? It is the basic skills that are needed to integrate our whole being into a well-conditioned whole. Setting up the ground floor is your entry level or pre-pilates work. Every person starts here, works through learning how to climb up without compromising their being as a whole. I will give you 12 essential steps to the holistic approach to well-being using Pilates:

1. Pilates equals posture – Become aware. How do you walk, stand and sit?

2. Alignment – is what feels right and what is right from your feet up?

3. Neutral spine and neutral pelvis – Finding it in your own body.

4. Pelvic floor and core activation – Do you feel those muscles work and do you know how to engage them properly?

5. Breathing – The importance of being present and connected to natural movement.

6. Control – the economy of movement, so each exercise has only

a few reps using only necessary muscles and effort for each movement.

7. Whole body Integration – Pilates exercises are always performed using the whole body.

8. Precision – is exact and intentional movement and is necessary to correct form.

9. Rhythm – is promoted by breathing to find natural movement and stimulates muscles to greater activity.

10. Centering – is the way the body is organized to move.

11. Balanced Muscle development – allows efficient movement and proper joint mechanics.

12. Concentration – is required to fully develop the body.

The mind and body must actively engage to achieve physical fitness. The Pilates philosophy and vision of health and well-being gives context to his exercises from his books, *Your Health*, 1934 and *Return to Life*, 1945. The Pilates method was created by Joseph H. Pilates. He was intuitive; he understood the body and designed specialized equipment that was innovative. He knew his work and vision of healthy living was "50 years ahead of (his) time." He developed the system of over 600 exercises of physical and mental conditioning for the various pieces of apparatus he invented. The Pilates equipment is designed to condition the entire body. Each piece of apparatus helps correct the body alignment and balance by simulating movements of functional activities. The exercise system starts from Pre-Pilates, beginner, intermediate, advanced and super-advanced can be performed on each apparatus as well as on the floor known as Mat work.

In our daily life, our busy days require us to find an intelligent exercise option. The mind-body discipline of Pilates has more than twelve million practitioners and is being taught all over the world. If you think about most exercise systems, they all have the ground floor foundation of the workout - which is Pilates based. It's good to know that every time I read a published or research-based article about flat abs, lower back care, athletic performance of sport teams, rehabilitation for injuries, celebrity workouts, Pilates is mentioned.

My clients come in looking for a change from their ordinary experiences of exercise and how to improve their body image, tone, and function. I give them the re-education of their body, mind and spirit. They learn about their body, posture, movement mechanics and how to maintain the body position and alignment. One of the most interesting parts is teaching a person how to breathe properly, it is so important and often ignored. "Breathing is the first act of life, and the last…above all learn how to breathe correctly." J.H. Pilates wrote in *Return to life through Contrology*, 1945. *Breathing* is a very normal function that is coordinated to be always present. We learn about how it affects our physical well-being and improves our movement patterns.

When I first meet with a person, the body is assessed through a postural assessment. This allows me to see any deviations from optimal alignment. Once I find what the ideal alignment looks like, I then design a program that would specifically be appropriate for that body. Have you ever noticed that not one body is the same? We may have similar body types, shapes and sizes, but there is not one person who is identically alike with another. I can give you a simple entry level to start understanding your own body, improve your own mind-body connection using the Pilates method. Many people sense an instant improved body awareness and image after the first session. They stand taller, look slimmer and have a greater sense of their own body alignment and posture than prior to the first visit. In this process of refinement, Pilates can change the body as a whole. Pilates can enhance every aspect of life when it is used to the full potential. It is one of the few exercise systems that can be adaptable for anyone and everyone. So if you want to look and feel better, or someone who wants to be pain free and able to function at optimal level, start now with the 12 steps.

Currently, I am a 2nd Generation Pilates Teacher designated from Lolita San Miguel in 2012. She is my mentor, a 1st Generation Pilates Teacher also known as a Pilates Elder. Ms. Miguel is one of the two people who were ever certified by Joseph H. Pilates to teach his method. I am also inspiring others to become Pilates teachers. I am honored to not only be an educator and presenter for Balanced Body, but my studio, Gold Coast Pilates LLC is Long Island's only Balanced Body® Authorized Training Center for Pilates and Barre Instructor Training and Continuing Education Courses.

I am living my dream now in my brand new fully-equipped studio which I relocated in Setauket, NY in 2010 – from where I started in my business in my home teaching clients while my children, ages 9 and 7, were infants. I have grown from one Instructor (myself) to nine Instructors while expanding the studio from 1,100 sq. feet to 3,200 sq. feet in April of 2013. My Certified staff is hand-selected, they bring their own personal expertise and are mentored by me. My goal is to give every Instructor, student, client and person my personal best. It is the knowledge, enthusiasm, and dedication to share this passion I have of Pilates. Every moment that I guide them to change a persons life as it has changed mine, brings me joy to have this honor to do so.

I am learning what Mr. Pilates meant by " The acquirement and enjoyment of physical well-being, mental calm and spiritual peace are priceless to their possessors if there be any such so fortunate living among us today. However, it is the ideal to strive for, and in our opinion, it is only through Contrology (Pilates) that this unique trinity of balanced body, mind, and spirit can ever be attained." ~ Joseph H. Pilates, in *Return to Life Through Contrology*, 1945.

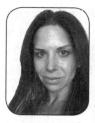

About Tattiana

Tattiana Gandolfo is the director and owner of Gold Coast Pilates LLC. She believes in whole body health and the way it integrates in our daily lives by creating wellness and longevity.

Tattiana is a 2nd Generation Pilates Teacher. She was designated a "Pilates Master Teacher" and "2nd Generation Pilates Teacher" under the mentorship of Lolita San Miguel, a "1st Generation Pilates Teacher/ Distinguished Elder" who was certified by Joseph H. and Clara Pilates. Tattiana was selected to be one of the few in the world who were mentored by Lolita San Miguel and successfully completed and graduated from the Lolita San Miguel, Pilates Master Mentor Program (PMMP) in December of 2011.

Tattiana is also comprehensively Certified by Polestar Pilates® Practitioner of Studio/Rehab, and a NASM® Certified Personal Trainer since 2003. She became a Faculty member and Presenter of Balanced Body® in 2009. She joins Balanced Body® as a Master Pilates Educator, training future Pilates Instructors and presenting continuing education courses. In August of 2012, Tattiana was privileged to be one of the first Balanced Body Barre Instructors who was taught by it's founder, Zayna Gold of Boston Body Pilates. In spring of 2013, Tattiana became also one of the first Balanced Body Barre Faculty and Presenters.

Tattiana provides her knowledge from a multitude of backgrounds. A former dancer and soccer player since the age of 4, Tattiana continued her passion for movement and the arts with figure skating, martial arts, weight training, yoga, a fashion and fitness model during her teens and later. She graduated *magna cum laude* from C.W. Post, Long Island University, with a B.F.A in the Performing and Visual Arts, and received the "Award for Excellence." Tattiana discovered Pilates in 2001 after suffering injuries and learned from her physical therapist about how Pilates exercises help, strengthen and prevent injury.

In 2005, Tattiana opened her own Pilates studio in her home, based on all of her training experiences in Scientific (Rehabilitation), Classical and Contemporary Pilates. She moved from her home studio in 2010 to her first commercial 1,100 sq. ft. location with two Pilates Instructors. In 2013, Gold Coast Pilates had expanded to 3,200 sq. ft., offering two group classrooms for Barre and Pilates equipment classes and a fully-equipped studio for Private training with a hand-picked and mentored staff of nine Instructors. She brought Balanced Body Barre to Long Island and currently teaches classes, individuals, mentors up and coming Instructors, and presents Pilates and Barre instructor trainings. Tattiana is always acquiring knowledge and sharing hers. In 2014, she was selected as one of America's PremierExperts and is co-authoring a book, *Rapid Body Makeover*, with John Spencer Ellis.

You can connect with Tattiana at:
tvg@goldcoastpilates.com
www.facebook.com/goldcoastpilates
www.twitter.com/goldcoastpilate
www.pinterest.com/goldcoastpilate
www.goldcoastpilates.com
www.thegoldbarre.com

CHAPTER 8

4 NUTRITIONAL MISTAKES PEOPLE MAKE WHEN TRYING TO SHED BODY FAT

BY NICK OSBORNE

Welcome to my chapter on having a nutritional plan. A proper nutritional plan (Not DIET!) is important in the quest for a better body, but most people have a ton of questions and are extremely confused by the amount of information that is out there.

Most of the information available is contradictory and designed to sell a product. I'm providing you simple but effective information to help you eat normal foods and achieve great results.

People don't realize that half of the results for a healthier body come from proper nutrition. Some people will say their goal is to add lean muscle, increase sport performance or just improve life. However, what people are after is fat loss.

This section is focused on fat loss rather than weight loss. Though everyone says they want weight loss, in reality, what they really want is to lose the layer of fat in between their organs and underneath their skin in order to feel better and look better. Weight loss can mean many things and some of them aren't even healthy.

It has been proven by science and also in my gym, *GO: Fitness Center*, that up to 91% of every pound of weight lost can be attributed to losing fat. This means that you're healthier and look better at the end of trying to lose 20 pounds of fat than you are if you don't make the four mistakes below.

Think about it. Your friend diets and loses 20 pounds but only loses between six and 10 pounds of fat. You use good nutrition and lose 20 pounds, 18 of which are fat. Which one of you is going to be happier, feel better and look better?

Where do the other pounds come from? It's usually from muscle and other tissues that your body needs to be healthy. That's why you need to think fat loss, not weight loss.

Another benefit to the fat loss from your nutrition plan is it enhances your mental and emotional well-being in addition to the physical changes. Proper nutrition and losing body fat will make you feel more in control of yourself, give you more confidence, and help your brain to function better.

MISTAKE #1
YOU DON'T HAVE A GOOD PLAN
WITHOUT A TIMELINE

To be successful with any endeavor, you need an effective plan with a clear goal and timeline. Most people just want to lose some weight, but they don't put a number on it or give it a timeframe (i.e., lose 20 pounds of fat in 18 weeks).

Since there is no plan and no timeline, they fail. Let's look at a realistic amount that you can lose.

Here are two different women's body types, weight loss and fat content:

	Woman #1	Woman #2
Body Weight:	150 lb.	180 lb.
Body Fat %:	20%	36%

Lean Body Mass: 120 lb.   115 lb.

Fat Body Mass: 30 lb.   65 lb.

As you can see, Woman #1 has more lean muscle and bone than Woman #2 but much less body fat. This means she is stronger, has more endurance, is healthier, and more than likely has a better self-image than the other woman.

So how does Woman #2 lose 31 pounds of fat as quickly and safely as possible? She would follow this plan...

Here are equations to figure out her (your) BMR:

Men:

66 + (6.3 x weight in pounds) + (12.9 x height in inches) - (6.8 x age in years) = Approximate BMR

Women:

655 + (4.3 x weight in pounds) + (4.7 x height in inches) - (4.7 x age in years) = Approximate BMR

Woman #2 = 655 + (4.3 x 180) + (4.7 x 66) - (4.7 x 32) = _____ Approx. BMR

655 + (774) + (310) - (150) = 1,589 BMR Calories

BMR w/ Activity Factor: *(how many calories you need for non exercise life)*

Multiply your BMR by your non-workout activity factor that most closely suits your lifestyle:

- *Sedentary - none or very little Mental and/or Physical Stress =   BMR X 1.2*

- *Light - Physical Stress (average of 3-4 days/week) = BMR X 1.375*

- *Moderate - Mental and/or Physical Stress (5 days/week) = BMR X 1.5*

> • *High - Mental and/or Physical Stress levels (more than 6+ days/week) = BMR X 1.7*

Approx. BMR:_____ x Activity Factor: _____ = Daily Calories to maintain current weight _____

Woman #2 *= Approx. BMR: 1,589 x Activity Factor: 1.2 = Daily Calories to maintain current weight = 1,907*

For Woman #2 to lose 1.2 pounds of fat a week the correct way, she must lose half of the fat from exercise and the other half from a nutritional plan.

This means reducing her calorie intake by approximately 375-400 calories per day, while eating the right foods at the right time and in the right amounts.

> *Daily Calories to maintain current weight _____ calories - 390 calories = _____ Daily Modified Calories to lose 1.5 pound per week*

> *Daily Calories for woman #2 to maintain current weight*

> *1,907 calories - 390 calories = 1,517 Daily Modified Calories to lose 1.5 pound per week*

>> • *Women should not go under 1,300 calories for health and safety reasons.*

>> • *Men should not go under 1,600 calories for health and safety reasons.*

Woman #2 should be eating 3 meals of approximately 375 calories and 3 snacks around 125 calories. This will keep her metabolism up and feeling full all day long.

She then needs to burn more than 2,600 calories a week from muscle building/metabolic workouts. (Getting on a treadmill 6 days a week WON'T work.)

This means Woman # 2 can lose 31 pounds of fat in approximately 26 weeks. It's completely doable while not turning into a workout and diet extremist.

To become more aware of what you're eating, you need to track it. The best way to do this is to get a notebook that fits in your pocket, and carry it with you while you're on your nutritional plan. Everything you put into your mouth, you will write down. This makes you hyper-aware of every time you throw a piece of candy or a cookie in your mouth, and shows you where your stumbling blocks are.

MISTAKE #2
YOU USE FOOD FOR MORE THAN FUEL

Here's a simple question. Would you be insulted if I or anyone else called you a dog? So, then why do you treat yourself like you would a dog? Think about it. You ask your dog to sit, he sits, and you give him a treat. While your dog is sitting, you ask him to shake and he raises his paw. In return, you give him a treat to reward and train him.

What do you think you do by treating yourself or rewarding yourself with food?

This isn't so bad if you see food as fuel for your body and you have great control over your cravings, emotions, and other excuses for overeating.

Some people look at food as a way to alleviate boredom. There has been a lot of research done, and anecdotal evidence given, that shows that a vast majority of people eat when they are bored, not just when they are hungry. Food ends up being a form of entertainment.

Another thing that children learn and carry over to adulthood is that when something good or bad goes on in our lives, we eat to celebrate or to reduce emotional pain.

Emotional eating is characteristic of somebody who is overweight. It is a vicious cycle. You overeat because you're not happy. You're unhappy because you are overweight. As a result, you go to the one thing that comforts you when you're unhappy…food. Often, we do this with our friends by going out to dinner or over-indulging in alcohol (we'll talk about this in a bit) to reduce our emotional pain.

If this is you and you can't get control of your eating, you might need help from a friend or even a counselor. However, being aware of emotional eating or eating out of boredom can change your actions.

It wouldn't be so bad if every time you had an emotional need to eat, you would go and binge on some celery and broccoli. However, that's not usually the case.

If you're tracking your eating, not only can you track what foods you are putting in your mouth, but also when you want to eat because of emotions, boredom or rewarding yourself. This awareness and tracking on a daily basis will go a long way in reversing unhealthy habits.

MISTAKE #3
CONSUMING ALCOHOL WHEN TRYING TO LOSE FAT

One question that comes up for many dieters is whether or not alcohol can be included in their diet plan. Alcohol is something that most adults do like to enjoy from time to time. So, what's the real deal about alcohol and your progress? Is this something that you can make room for in your diet or is it something that you need to give the boot?

When alcohol arrives at the liver, it's tagged as being a toxin and the body works to eliminate it as quickly as possible. The liver converts the alcohol into something called acetate. The body then looks to burn this acetate before any other energy sources in order to get rid of it.

This is very important from a fat loss perspective. While your body is working to burn this acetate for fuel to get rid of it quickly, other energy sources like fat and carbs get put in a "holding pattern." In essence, while you're working to burn off the alcohol, the burning of fat for fuel gets put on hold. You CANNOT burn fat in the presence of alcohol!

You need to be aware of how many calories are actually in alcohol. Alcohol contains seven calories per gram, whereas both proteins and carbs contain just four. Fat comes in at the highest calorie value per gram at nine, which places alcohol right in the middle.

However, alcohol is often mixed with other things. If you're drinking your alcohol with high calorie or high fat mixers such as cream, sodas, or sugary mixers, you could easily end up with a drink that packs in well over 300 calories per serving.

If you take in three or four of these over the course of a night, the calories add up fast. Plus, don't believe the low calorie beer myth. The government only counts alcohol as having 4 calories per gram, not 7. Sneaky, eh? So, you're consuming more calories than you realize.

It doesn't stop there. Alcohol actually stimulates hunger. If you're eating a meal with an alcoholic beverage, you may be full from your meal but when you continue to consume alcohol, you will continue to overeat. There are no fat calories in alcohol but it has high caloric content. Your body will use this as its source of energy but will store all other nutrients as body fat.

Another issue with alcohol is missing meals. Many people skip meals because they know they're going out drinking. This is horrible. When you skip a meal, you're slowing down your metabolism and setting yourself up for body fat storage. On top of that, the alcohol you consume is loaded with calories.

If you want to be truly successful with your fat loss and workout program, it's best if you can forgo alcohol for the time being. One drink every now and then may not hurt but if you're taking in any more than this, it will definitely hinder your progress.

MISTAKE #4
NOT EATING REAL FOOD AND BEING SOLD ON SUPPLEMENTS

Hopefully, the big supplement companies don't read this chapter, because I'm going to tell you that you don't need what they're selling in most cases.

The only supplement that I recommend for my clients is a good multivitamin. Understand, the word supplement means "to add to" or "in addition to." Not to replace. You have to eat right first, before adding supplements. Supplements DON'T replace a good nutrition plan.

This means that in good nutrition plans, you have to learn how to eat real foods. That way, when you are at a restaurant, staying with friends, or having to make choices, you aren't restricted to one company's definition of what food is.

In addition, some "fat loss supplements" actually stress your body and could cause you to gain more body fat over time once you go back to eating normal foods.

Most supplements contain some sort of stimulant. Either caffeine, ephedra, synephrine, or something of this nature. These stimulants make your body remain under physical stress for an extended period of time. This will result in a rise of adrenaline and cortisol. Cortisol is the hormone that makes your body want to store fat.

Learning to eat real food, prepared in a healthy way, and learning to eat a combination of protein, fibrous carbs, and starchy carbs in the morning, as well as not eating starchy carbs in the afternoon and evening is key to your success.

Protein powders, bars, meal replacement shakes and other "healthy snacks" should only be used if needed to supplement your nutritional plan because of convenience. In other words, if you're at your desk and need a protein shake and an apple for a snack, because bringing in a chicken breast for a snack is inconvenient, that's understandable. However, having five protein shakes a day isn't.

Diet drinks aren't any better than their sugary counterparts. These drinks have chemicals that have been proven to be dangerous. I'm not going to go into the debate of what levels are acceptable risks and what are not, but if something is not healthy in large doses, it's probably not healthy in small doses either. If you need to flavor your water, let cucumbers, strawberries, or other fruits soak in your water overnight to give it a slight flavor. Drinking as much purified water as possible each day is going to keep you healthy, increase your metabolism, speed up your recovery, and help you burn body fat.

Another thing about consuming diet drinks and diet foods is that your brain is expecting something sweet when you eat these foods.

Your brain runs on carbohydrates. When you tease your brain that you are going to give it something sweet, because your tongue detects sweetness, but your brain does not receive an increase in sugars, it feels cheated, and will increase your cravings.

At this point, you're going to start craving more and more foods with sugars/starch in them. Since your self-control is just like a muscle, it will get fatigued over time. If you're drinking two or three cans of diet pop during the day and your brain is not getting the sugars, your self-control is getting fatigued and you end up binging at 7 or 9 o'clock... right before you go to bed.

It's much better to fill up on real, clean food, and not tease your brain or body with fake sugars, giving you more stress and more frustration.

TO FINISH UP

You need to make sure that you're developing a plan for your nutrition program that is going to:

- Keep you from failing

- Keep you on track

- Be realistic for your life

- Include real foods

- Help you reach your goal in the time you need

- AND keep you from being frustrated and unhappy

If you can do this, you're going to be able to reach your goals faster than you thought, while feeling good, gaining self-confidence, and being in more control of yourself than ever before.

1,500 Calories Per Day Nutrition Plan

Ultra Clean & Simple

BREAKFAST

1/2 cup	Uncooked Quick Oatmeal	149 Cal.
6 oz.	Fat Free - Flavored Yogurt	150 Cal.

SNACK 1

1/2 Serving	Protein Drink	125 Cal.
2	Plain Rice Cakes	70 Cal.

LUNCH

5 oz.	Chicken Breast	155 Cal.
1 Cup	Steamed Rice	180 Cal.

SNACK 2

1 Slices	Grain Bread	80 Cal.
1 TBL.	Peanut Butter	95 Cal.

DINNER

4 oz.	Broiled Salmon	232 Cal.
1	Medium Salad	75 Cal.
2 tbl	Light Oil & Vinegar Dressing	40 Cal.

SNACK 3

1/2 Serving	Protein Drink	125 Cal.

On The Go

BREAKFAST

1/2	Cinnamon Bagel	78 Cal.
1/4	Cantaloupe	47 Cal.
1 1/2 Cup	1% Milk	150 Cal.

SNACK 1

1 Cup	Strawberries	49 Cal.
1/2 cup	Cottage Cheese - 1% fat	82 Cal.

LUNCH

1 Serving	Wendy's® Jr. Hamburger	270 Cal.
1 Serving	Wendy's® Small Chili	200 Cal.

SNACK 2

1	Hard Boiled Egg	78 Cal.
6 oz.	V-8® Vegetable Juice - No Salt	50 Cal.

DINNER

1/2 cup	Whole Wheat Spaghetti	85 Cal.
1/2 cup	Marinara Sauce	110 Cal.
3	Lean Turkey Meatballs	150 Cal.

SNACK 3

4"	Banana	53 Cal.
1 Cup	1% Milk	100 Cal.

Figure 1

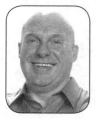

About Nick

Nick Osborne has been in the fitness industry for more than 25 years. He's been a part of every aspect of the gym business from desk person, membership sales person and head personal trainer; …all the way to owner of two clubs.

He has seen all the fads come and go. He focuses on building systems and methods that get people fast results, in a fun and effective way. He created his gyms to be the most effective training gyms in the Columbus, Ohio area, by providing fun workouts and training his coaches up to 12 times longer than any of his competitors.

The secret to his gym's success is not just the effective and fun exercise systems, but more so how the coaches/trainers and staff work with and treat the members. His coaches focus on every aspect of the clients' lives that can affect them getting the results they want. His systems also provide nutrition education, cardio workouts and metabolic circuit training, as well as foam rolling and stretching programs to each and every coaching client.

Nick's system is so effective for the club, coach/trainer and client that fitness centers around the world have sought him out for consulting, public speaking and to implement his system into their own gyms. Nick has become the "Trainer of Personal Trainers."

Nick used his "Integrated Functional Coaching System®" (IFCS) to train himself to win 14 U.S. titles in full-contact and traditional Kung Fu, and a World Championship in Traditional Combat Kung Fu. Also, he is the only person to win N.A.S.S.'s North America's Strongest Man twice.

The IFCS has also been used in training professional athletes, World's Strongest Man champion, Phil Pfister, The Ohio State University varsity football, wrestling and field hockey teams, as well as guiding more than 100,000 people around the world to get the bodies they want.

To learn more about Nick Osborne and his training center, you can visit the gym's website: www.GoFitnessCenter.com or call 614-481-8080.

CHAPTER 9

FUNK'S FIVE SECRETS TO SUPERCHARGE YOUR METABOLISM AND SCULPT A LEAN, MUSCULAR BODY

BY FUNK ROBERTS

Remember when we were young and could eat and drink anything we wanted and still stay lean? Or perhaps you knew someone, that no matter what he/she ate they would never put on a pound. That used to be me. In my late teens and early 20's, I could eat anything I wanted and still stay shredded. Why?

Well, at the time I was really active as a professional volleyball player. I was pretty muscular too which helped to keep my metabolism super high. That used to frustrate all my friends and family with the amount of food I could eat and not look any different.

But as I got older, and after retiring from playing pro volleyball in my early thirties, my life started to change with the typical 9 to 5 jobs, daily activities and kids. I ballooned up from a ripped 185 lbs. to 215lbs of what is called Male PMS (Puffy Muscle Syndrome). Even though I was in the gym six days a week, training for up to two hours, I was big and soft with a spare tire.

It all changed after one day while I was training with a friend and he said to me, "Doesn't it upset you that you invest so much time in the gym and your body really hasn't changed? You would think by now you'd be pretty ripped." But I wasn't...and what he said stuck with me for a while. That was the turning point for me.

I began my research to find most effective ways to workout and eat so that I can get the lean, ripped and muscular physique. When I found and implemented these methods/tricks I'm about to share with you, my body instantly changed.

In fact, within 6 months I was lean ripped and back down to 185lbs! I started to share these tricks with my personal training clients, boot campers and they all got amazing results.

If you use the following simple tricks, I guarantee that you can quickly boost your metabolism and incinerate stubborn fat faster than you ever thought possible.

Let's go over what you need to know:

Metabolism is your Fat Burning Monster

Before I start, it important that you understand what your metabolism is in the first place and why it slows down.

Your metabolic rate is how many calories your body burns off per day to stay alive. This means keeping your lungs functioning, the digestive system working and your heart beating.

All the physical activity you do throughout the day gets added to your basal metabolic rate, and then you have your total daily calorie burn.

Your metabolism also has a lot to do with what you eat and more importantly how much muscle you have. The more muscle a person has, the more calories it takes to maintain.

As we get older our metabolism seems to slow down. But according to the Mayo Clinic, the illusion that your metabolism slows as you age actually occurs because as you get older, your muscle mass decreases and your amount of fat tends to increase.

Our lives change significantly as we get older.

We have much more responsibility and find ourselves spending more time on long commutes to work, hours in an office chair and busy with family or kids. The point is that we definitely move a lot less now than we did when we were younger – especially if you have kids.

But I have good news for you today! In fact, it's great news!

Isn't it awesome to know that a person indeed has a lot of control over their metabolism? Aging is not a death sentence for metabolism. On the contrary, most of a person's metabolism can be controlled through these tricks that I'm about to share with you.

So I am now going to share with you my 5 tricks that will help increase your metabolism so you can burn fat, build lean muscle and stay lean all year round.

TRICK #1 – EMBRACE THE POWER OF METABOLIC TRAINING

— Metabolic Training and how it will help you burn fat and build lean muscle

The short definition of metabolic training is completing compound exercises with little rest in between in an effort to maximize calorie burn and increase metabolic rate during and after the workout.

Unlike traditional weight-training routines, which exercise isolated muscle groups one at a time, compound exercises target multiple joints and muscles concurrently. Only this method will raise your metabolism, burn fat and develop lean, dense muscle mass each and every day.

Metabolic training is high intensity anaerobic exercise that makes you breathless. An example would be a circuit where you would perform as many reps as you can of an exercise for a brief period lasting 15 to 60 seconds with rest periods of 15 to 30 seconds. It's basically high intensity intervals followed by low intensity intervals.

This type of training is set up to increase your work capacity, which is the ability to perform an amount of work in a specified period of time. The more work you can do in a shorter period of time, the more power you will produce.

Power is a key element to getting a lean, fit body as power production triggers the natural release of Human Growth Hormone (HGH). HGH metabolizes fat for energy that your body uses for muscle growth. Simply stated, you lose fat while gaining dense muscle. HGH also enhanced protein synthesis in your muscles making them stronger and larger. Ladies, please don't worry...you will never bulk up on this program unless you choose to use steroids. This is not something I endorse.

In summary, higher intensity begets you more power. Increased power equals more HGH. The higher the production of HGH the more your body will metabolize fat and increase muscle mass. And muscle increases your metabolism and burns fat!

It's time to stop using traditional weight training and start implementing metabolic workout into your overall regimen.

TRICK #2 – BENEFIT FROM THE "AFTERBURN EFFECT"

Another way to increase your metabolism is by tapping into the "afterburn effect".

The use of metabolic circuits trigger the "afterburn effect" which will help you burn fat for up to **36 hours after you're finished**. This uses a concept called excess post-exercise oxygen consumption (EPOC). This is a phenomenon that occurs any time you've performed extremely intense exercise where you alternate very brief periods of all-out exercise lasting 15 to 60 seconds with active rest periods two to three times as long.

This relates to what is called EPOC or Excess Post-Exercise Oxygen Consumption.

In other words, after a metabolic workout your body's metabolism is very high.

Basically, because you are resting at this time, your body is tapping into the fat stores for energy through oxygen. Oxygen burns fat.

Your body takes a lot longer to recover after metabolic workouts; therefore your body is burning fat for a longer period. Science shows that metabolic workouts place such an intense demand on the system that it takes your body up to 36 hours to work its way back to homeostasis (a normal state).

This is essentially how much additional energy the body burns off above and beyond the calories burned off during the workout session in order to recover properly. This literally turns you into a calorie and fat-incinerating furnace, even if you're just lying on the couch or enjoying YouTube.

On the flip side, after a long and boring 45-60 minutes duration on the elliptical or exercise machine at the gym, because you are not exercising at high level (per se), your EPOC or post-workout metabolism is not that high nor does it last very long.

So it's time to substitute long boring cardio sessions for metabolic circuits – so that you can tap into the afterburn effect (EPOC) 24 to 36 hours after you are done.

TRICK #3 – PROTEIN POWER!

Next, it's absolutely essential that you have enough protein in your diet. Protein is a powerful food, and by ensuring that you eat a source of protein with each meal and snack, you will feel full longer, build more muscle and even burn fat.

Proteins are primarily used as our body's building blocks. Protein is needed for muscle growth and repair. Basically, proteins are made up of long chains of amino acids. There are 22 different types of amino acids and the body needs all of them to function properly. Amino acids provide the raw material for building proteins in the body. However, unlike carbohydrates and fats, amino acids are not stored in the body, therefore requiring you to constantly replenish their supply in order to make new protein.

Eating protein is a great way to increase your metabolism because of its thermogenic – metabolic properties (TEF - Thermic Effect of Feeding), which is the amount of energy your body expends to chew, swallow and digest food. Protein has a high thermic effect from eating. This means your body uses more energy just to digest protein, so the more protein you eat, the more energy you burn (less food stored as fat).

The body will actually expend a large number of calories just breaking that protein down, therefore increasing your total daily calorie burn.

After eating protein, your metabolic rate will increase by approximately 30 percent. In other words, if you eat 100 calories of protein, 30 of those will be burned just digesting and using the protein. By comparison, the thermic effect of carbohydrates is typically around 10 percent, and fat is just 5 percent.

For those of you that like numbers, aim to eat 1.4 to 2 grams of protein per kilogram of body weight (or roughly 0.6 to 0.9 grams per pound of bodyweight). For an 80 kg person, this would mean trying to eat around 112 to 160 grams per day.

High quality protein sources include fish, chicken, turkey, lean beef, eggs (and egg whites), Greek yogurt, cottage cheese, protein supplements (e.g., whey protein powder).

By reading this section you should have learned that the key to this trick is to ensure that you are eating a source of protein with each meal and snack as it will help you build more muscle, stay fuller longer, and even burn more fat because protein is more thermogenic - metabolic (TEF).

TRICK #4 – GET YOUR CARBS ON!

Are you on a low carb diet? If so, you probably think you're on your way to rapid fat loss. But you're wrong.

While low carb diets can promote quick weight loss, there's one caveat. Low carb diets can dramatically slow the metabolic rate as a hormone called leptin starts to decrease. As it decreases, your urge to eat will get stronger and stronger until it's eventually not tolerable any longer.

You'll be able to take total control of your metabolism and maximize fat loss if you consume your carbs from starches and fruits in your post-workout anabolic window of opportunity. Simply stated, up to an hour after a high intensity, metabolic training session is the best time for your starchy carbs.

After a metabolic training session your body has depleted its glycogen stores. These stores need replenishing so your body doesn't hold fat as energy storage for later. Your body will use the carbs IMMEDIATELY for energy, which will prevent it from dipping into your muscles for energy.

There have been multiple clinical studies by top universities proving the most important 60 minutes of the day to make your body burn the most fat and calories than it otherwise would, is within the first hour after finishing your workout!

They all concur that within this "Golden Hour", you should consume a meal or shake with a minimum 2 to 1 mixture of fast-absorbing carbohydrates, high-concentration proteins and certain other nutrients. 4:1 is optimal if you are performing an extremely high metabolic workout, however 2:1 or 3:1 is acceptable.

If your body does not get the nutrients it needs right after your workout, you are flushing a lot of your exercise efforts down the drain. In addition to this, without this practice you will weaken your fat-burning metabolism, lose muscle, suffer more pain, have more fatigue and your performance will suffer the next time you workout. WOW!

After the workout, your body is in the state of catabolism and starving for the carbohydrates and protein that it needs to recover and repair.

This meal will start the recovery process quicker and keeps your fat-burning metabolism going.

During this state, your muscles will absorb nutrients much like a sponge would water since your glycogen stores are drastically diminished. The carbs will be used by your body to restore the glycogen.

Imagine you didn't have the post-workout carbs; what would your body do? It will look within to find energy and breakdown muscle tissue instead. Not a good thing!

Bottom line, if you are looking for the best way to refuel your body after a metabolic training session, then make sure you eat your starchy carbs after (at least 2:1 or 3:1 ratio of carbohydrate to protein). Eat within one hour after your training session for optimal fat loss, lean muscle development and overall performance.

TRICK #5 – STAY CONSISTENT.

One of the most effective ways to continually burn fat and build lean muscle is to be consistent and follow through.

You can have the best program on the planet, you can have a sure-fire nutrition plan and you can have a gut-wrenching determination, but if you are not consistent, your results will always be sub-par at best. In fact it is so important that I will tell you right now without reservation that your success will depend almost completely on how consistent you are.

Staying consistent is the only way to reap the rewards of your hard work. Results in weight loss don't come in the blink of an eye, they take time but they do come. Did you put the excess weight on in two weeks? Of course you didn't! What makes you think you can take it off in two weeks?

Most people give up after a couple of weeks because they are impatient and expect too much too soon. STAY THE COURSE!!! Once you get past the first two months, you will begin to see significant results, and after that, the results will come quicker and quicker. The longest wait is in the beginning but don't give up.

Maintain your consistent drive to succeed and follow your program every step of the way!

So there you have the five tricks that you can use to increase your metabolic rate and finally burn that stubborn fat from your body while building lean muscle. I promise that if you implement even just a few of these into your program plan, you will start to notice a dramatic difference.

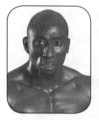

About Funk

Funk Roberts, President and Creator of Funk Roberts Fitness, is a former Professional Beach Volleyball player turned Fitness trainer. Funk is an online fat loss expert that helps thousands of people worldwide burn unwanted fat while building lean muscle through his website, videos, articles, media and fitness products.

Funk is a Certified Metabolic Training Expert, Kettlebell Specialist, Mixed Martial Arts Conditioning Coach, TRX Qualified, Celebrity Fat Loss Expert and Certified Personal Trainer. He was just named one of America's Premier Experts and has been seen on ABC, NBC, CBS and Fox TV Affiliates in the summer of 2013.

Funk has been a featured trainer in a few fitness training DVD's and has produced his own online products such as: *Elite Strength and Conditioning for Combat Athletes, Funk's 6 Week Jump Training Program* and the newly-launched *Spartan Training System 10 Week Fat Loss Program.*

Funk is passionate about helping people transform their body and educating them on how to lead a healthy lifestyle. His mission is to help 500,000 people by 2014 change their life's using fitness, nutrition and motivation.

His more than 30 years of training, expertise, research and experience has made the difference in helping others change their lives for the better. Funk has a following of over 40,000 subscribers to his websites, along with 58,000 YouTube subscribers and over 200,000 fans on Facebook, and he communicates with them on a daily-to-weekly basis.

He continues to learn and improve his skills so that he can supply the best information and contribute to the fitness community and help people make a difference in their lives.

At a young 45-year-old, Funk is married and has 2 older children. His passion is training men, women, teens and athletes, helping people transform their lives, traveling and spending time with his wife and family.

CHAPTER 10

SEVEN

BY EAMONN DEANE

7 STEPS TO LOSING 7 POUNDS IN 7 DAYS!

This chapter and the associated complimentary online resources mentioned within will provide you with the knowledge on how to jumpstart yourself to a healthier lifestyle, and finally get you on track to getting the body you desire. It is written in a simplified and easy-to-follow manner, with a focus on you having an enjoyable experience while achieving amazing results. The average weight loss for the seven days is seven pounds so this process can be very inspirational as well as rewarding. I will not only outline what to do but also WHY you should do it. I believe that if we understand why we are doing something then we are much more likely to follow through. Awareness precedes change.

The 7-day plan can be labeled a number of different things ranging from "kickstart" to "jumpstart" to the all-so-controversial word "detox".

I have often called it a detox or detoxification stage for a number of reasons, even though it is very different to 99% of detox diets out there. It consists of nutrient dense foods that fuel your body and help you reach optimal vitality. It is NOT a typical fad juice or shake-only diet.

Why should you follow it? It has been the start of a complete life and body transformation for thousands of people. When I started my online coaching journey, I had 1200 people join to take part in this seven-day program. I have run it many times since, with each group of participants ranging from 1,000 to 3,500. It's simple, effective and empowering.

Before I outline the guidelines for the 7 days, I will explain why the word detox can be controversial in the health and fitness industry and why those fad juice diets are the wrong path to choose.

Humans are amazing and highly intelligent creatures. Our bodies constantly assess and adapt to our surroundings and automatically function in a way that results in life. As you read this text, your brain and body are undergoing numerous functions. Your brain is signaling to your eyes to move from the top of the page to the bottom in typewriter fashion and then comprehend what you see and take in on the way down, your heart is pumping oxygenated blood to all of your working body systems, your lungs are removing harmful gases from your body and inhaling more oxygen, and your liver is digesting and absorbing nutrients from foods you have eaten. This list goes on and becomes much more detailed as these processes go down to the cellular level.

All of the above functions are essential for life and so your body and brain have figured out how to complete them. Certain body functions can be listed under a process called detoxification. So yes, your body detoxifies itself automatically. If it did not, then there would be no human life. And that's one reason why many of those detox diets are labeled fads. I mean, why detox if your body already does it for you, right? Here's a better question – How efficiently is your body detoxifying?

We live in a toxic environment and the western diet is one packed with processed foods and high in sugar, alcohol and caffeine. Many foods, liquids and chemicals can prevent some of our organs functioning correctly, which can lead to poor detoxification. If we aren't detoxing effectively, then it is much more difficult to lose fat. If we eliminate toxic foods, eat whole natural foods and provide the body with all of the nutrients it needs, then we can restore optimum functioning, which will aid the detoxification process. The liver is our primary detoxification organ and produces a number of important hormones. A healthy liver will result in a more vibrant fulfilling life and an accelerated rate of HEALTHY fat loss. What you will learn in this chapter may change your life and be the missing link you were looking for.

I have outlined the plan's main elements in seven easy-to-follow steps:

(1). Recovery

Sleep is our body's main method of recovery and repair, and is a limiting factor for a high percentage of people when it comes to achieving their goals. If you want to feel, look, think and perform better, then you need to assess your sleeping patterns and habits.

It is the general public's conception that once you get a certain amount of hours (usually 8) that you fulfilled your body's needs. But quality is just as important as duration. High quality sleep is essential for not only optimal fat loss and muscle building, but also health and vitality.

It's recommended that you sleep 6 to 8 hours a night and the best sleeping window is from approximately 10pm to 6am. 10pm to 2am is the optimal physiological (body) repair window and 2am to 6am is the optimal psychogenic (mind) repair window. Sleep outside of these windows will still result in repair and recovery, but isn't as effective.

The optimal 10 pm to 6 am window is formed as a result of our body clock or circadian rhythm – a naturally occurring 24 hour cycle that determines the sleeping patterns of humans and is closely linked to biological activity like hormone production, cell regeneration and brain wave activity. As sunlight goes down, our body produces less cortisol (a stress hormone). In the evening our testosterone begins to rise to prime our muscles for repair when we sleep. This increase in testosterone is at its peak at approximately 10 pm to 2 am. Any sleep interruptions in the physiological repair window, or if you miss half of it, then you are reducing your body's ability to repair its muscles effectively that you may have trained earlier during the day. Same principle goes for the psychogenic repair window. If you miss or have interruptions during that stage you may wake up feeling a lot more stressed than usual. Just ask someone that works irregular shifts or a mother to a newborn baby if they often feel run down, stressed and often lacking energy. YES! Our cells regenerate when we sleep. Give them the best opportunity you can and you will see huge benefits.

Some sleep tips to go along with this sleeping window:

- Black out your room and dim lights at night – Make your room as dark as possible and avoid any bright electronics like the laptop or television an hour before you sleep. Dim the room lights or use smaller lamps rather than a central bright light in the middle of the roof. Light, especially bright and blue, suppresses the production and release of melatonin. Melatonin is a hormone that is secreted into the blood at night and makes you feel less alert.

- Avoid caffeine after 10 am. Caffeine is a stimulant that will affect the quality of your sleep. If you need that morning pick me up, then a cup of black coffee is fine if taken before 10 am. For the rest of the day try green tea as a coffee replacement. And in the evening, tulsi tea is very good for helping people to wind down.

- Establish a pre-bed ritual – Take part in an activity that relaxes you 15-20 minutes before bed. An action packed horror movie just before bed will leave you stressed getting into bed. Instead try reading, yoga, having a bath or an activity that helps you wind down. And remember, do so in as little light as possible.

- Bed – Invest in a comfortable bed and don't use your phone as an alarm clock. Instead get a normal bedside alarm and leave your phone in a different room.

Try the above for the seven days and you will notice a difference. Getting sunlight/daylight soon after you wake will improve your cortisol awakening response, which will make the process become more natural and make you feel more alert in the mornings.

In the past I have experimented with clients and myself whereby the only variable we changed to our lifestyles was our sleeping routine, so current exercise patterns and nutritional habits remained the same. We did this for a weeklong period and the average weight loss was between 2-4 pounds just for improving quality of sleep. Our bodies were less stressed and therefore bodily functions like absorption, digestion, hormone production and suppression and cell regeneration were more effective – which therefore aided fat loss. Sleep is a very common limiting factor and could be what's holding you back.

(2). Hydration

Adequate water is ESSENTIAL for this program to work. Our body is primarily made up of water. Try drinking 3 liters a day other than your workout water (1 liter). If you don't drink enough water, you won't flush all of the toxins out of your system and you need water for all bodily functions. A good habit to get into is carrying around a bottle of water with you, as convenience will create fewer barriers to drinking a high quantity.

In the morning first thing after you wake, drink a half-liter of water with some added lemon juice and ginger root (half an inch). This will help alkalize your body and benefits the liver.

(3). Elimination

Keeping this section simple, we will be removing the following from the diet: gluten/wheat, dairy, processed foods, yogurt, sugar and alcohol. If possible, remove caffeine for the seven days but it is not essential. However as outlined in the first step, just have one cup of black coffee before 10 am. Remove all carbohydrates for the 7 days. All vegetables except for root vegetables will remain in the diet. All fruit except for berries should also be removed. I know it may sound crazy restricting fruit, but they are very high in sugar. Berries however are high in antioxidants so they are fine, but don't go overboard (a handful or two a day). Check the free online site to get a full list of foods to avoid for the week. Okay, so if we are removing all that, then you are probably wondering what is left to eat. Good question. Check the next step.

(4). Target

Okay, so you need to remove a few things from your diet. But what do you add and replace the foods you removed with? The answer is real fresh whole foods. NOT juices or shakes. This is NOT a typical fad, detox diet. You need to provide your body with the nutrients it needs. In general go for fresh and organic foods when possible and avoid highly processed foods. As a rule of thumb, the quicker a food spoils, the healthier it is for you, and if you can't pronounce certain ingredients on the packaging, then avoid it

You should eat 4 to 5 meals a day. These will include your three main meals, breakfast, lunch and dinner, and 1 to 2 snacks. If you don't have an active vocation or high intensity exercise plan, I would stick to three main meals and one snack. However, try this for the first two days and if you find yourself lacking energy throughout the day, then add a second snack.

Your three main meals should consist of a protein source, lots of green vegetables and a healthy fat source. [Check the extensive shopping list available for free online to see the different foods allowed]. The protein portion size should be similar to one palm of your hand for females and two palms for males. Green vegetables should take up approximately 60% of your plate, and the healthy fat source can be something like a handful of nuts, two tablespoons of cashew/almond nut butter, an avocado or another healthy fat source from the shopping list. While on the point of green vegetables, I really can't emphasize how important they are. The more cruciferous vegetables you eat, the easier this process will be and the better the result. The darker green and more leafy the vegetable, the better – 60% of each of your three main meals – but really there is no restriction for the 7 days on green leafy vegetables. For protein, any option from the shopping list is fine. Healthy fats also play a huge role. Don't neglect them.

(5). Supplementation

Supplements are optional for the 7 days but can be beneficial. The three baseline supplements I recommend are:

• Omega 3 fish oil – Purchase only omega 3 and not omega 3

combined with omega 6 and 9. The reason for this is that the omega 3 to omega 6 balances in the body should be 1:1. For most people it is around 1:15 due to processed foods among other things. Optimal fat loss and muscle building occurs when the ratio is closest to 1:1 due to hormone optimization. When purchasing the supplement look out for a high EPA/DHA level on the front of the container. You should aim to take around 1gram of EPA/DHA with each of your three main meals.

- Greens Drink – I suggest Wheatgrass. This will help alkalize your body. Due to the environment we live in we are constantly ingesting acidic foods we need to kick your body into a more alkaline environment. Fat cells thrive in acidic conditions and hate alkaline conditions. Get the powder form and take a teaspoon in a half-liter of water or take as a shot in the morning.

- L-glutamine – L-glutamine is excellent for gut health and muscle recovery. Your gut is also strongly linked with your brain. Every wonder why you get butterflies? The gut is often referred to as the second brain and it is extremely important for optimum brain function. If you think about it the brain is dependent on the nutrients from the digestion that occurs in the gut. The brain and gut are actually formed from the same clump of tissue and then they separate during foetal development. Nearly every hormone and neurotransmitter that controls the brain has been found in the gut.

- The gut is actually the main producer of neurotransmitters, which are responsible for our psychological state. 80% of serotonin (our "happy feel good" hormone) is produced in the gut. If you have poor gut health you are restricting how good you can feel everyday by almost 80%. If you are wise about the food you consume, then you will take care of your gut health. A healthy gut will then help regulate a better psychological state and promote a sense of well being and optimum brain function. You can get this in powder form and pill form. Try powder form and take a teaspoon each morning in a half a litre of water, or as a shot like the wheatgrass.

- Magnesium – Not one of my three baseline supplements, but magnesium is an often-ignored mineral that quite a few people are deficient in. Supplementing with magnesium oil spray can help improve sleep quality. The spray is better than the capsules due to the high absorption rates our skin is capable of.

- Other supplements like whey protein, vitamin D, ashwaganda are all beneficial, and I have information on each of those in the online resources.

(6). Exercise

For the 7 days, try and get in a mix of resistance training and suitable cardio or active recovery. A sample week may look like:

— Monday, Wednesday, Friday – Resistance training

— Tuesday, Thursday, Saturday – Suitable cardio or active recovery

For resistance training, it is best to incorporate bigger movements like squats, lunges, and shoulder presses. For active recovery you can do something like light cardio or yoga, and if you are advanced, you could do sprints instead. (Check the extensive online resources for a full sample.)

(7). Mindset, Habits and Strategies

It is very easy for me to advise you to think positively. However, I almost guarantee that you have most likely heard this advice numerous times already, and you know as well as I do that life can throw things at us that make it very difficult to only think positively all day, every day. Positive thinking is important and to be encouraged. However. this is not always possible, and the problem lies within the brain.

Our brain is made up of three main parts. First you have the "reptilian" or "animal" part, which is the first section of our brain to evolve and is solely focused on survival. Then we have the limbic system which is the emotional center of the brain, and finally the neo-cortex or "human" part of the brain, which is the final section to evolve. It is within the neo-cortex or human part of the brain that thinking takes place and logic thoughts occur. But we are not always in that part of our brain.

If you are in the human part of your brain, you will have no problem adhering to a nutrition program and having a positive mindset. In the human part, we are in response mode, which means before every action there is a thought process that will create a positive response. However, different types of stress and threats to our survival cause us to instantly move to and reside in our reptilian or animal brain. Once there, our focus is to survive, not thrive. Positive thinking and goal achievement is no longer on the priority list, but instead we enter reaction mode and react with animal instinct. When someone on a fat loss program decides to overeat or eat a lot of sugar, for example, it's not the human, it's the animal in them reacting to the desire for that food. The human would think logically about the complications of overeating and then decide it's best not to.

These animal reactions happen to everyone. If it weren't for the reaction mode of our animal brain, we would rarely escape real dangers when presented with them. What has happened to many people though, is that they are in reaction mode for too long. The good news is that this can be easily overcome by creating strategies to deal with certain stressful or challenging situations. Also awareness precedes change. Realizing why you do certain things is the first step to changing it. Create new habits to replace old, negative ones and introduce strategies (check online resource) that result in positive actions and allow for more positive thinking and self-empowerment.

I hope the information and guidelines given both in this chapter and the online resource site, provide you with the guidelines you need to reach your goal. Live the life you want. Break free from the one you don't.

— E.D.

Dedicated to Archie, George, and Isaac, and the Join Our Boys Trust

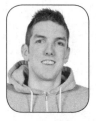

About Eamonn

Top health and fitness coach Eamonn Deane is currently recognized as an expert in the body and life transformation field – due to his ability to help anyone reach their goals and dreams through both online and offline coaching. From nutrition, exercise, holistic health and sport science all the way to life coaching qualifications, Eamonn has an array of knowledge that he loves to apply with his clients.

Having one of the most interesting and impressive business start-up stories, the Irish entrepreneur is taking the health and fitness world by storm, attracting clients from six continents just one month after he started his online business. Although Irish, Eamonn has been seen on American television networks NBC, ABC, CBS and Fox and has been requested to speak in America. When asked about his success story, he attributes it to his desire to invest in and educate himself, as well as the personal attention he gives to each of his clients.

Eamonn has such a love and passion for coaching that he never feels like he is at work. Some other activities he enjoys are travelling, training, skydiving, white water kayaking, playing the guitar, spending time with friends and playing with his dog, Rocky.

Eamonn's 10 year dream and vision is to build a foundation that gives seven figures a year to worthy causes, make a difference in the educational system by promoting more entrepreneurship and creativity, and make massive changes for the better in the health and fitness industry. Over the coming years, Eamonn wants to continue to change thousands of lives through his online and offline coaching business.

Website: www.eamonndeane.com
Facebook: www.facebook.com/eamonndeanefitness
Email: eamonn@eamonndeane.com

CHAPTER 11

ALL ABOUT YOU

BY DAVID OSGATHORP

The alarm clock blasts out again, the snooze button has been hit four times already this morning and you know it's now going to take record time for you to get ready and get out to work. You drag yourself from your bed and stumble across the room. Immediately you regret that bottle of wine that "had to be finished off" last night, as you make your way to the shower in an attempt to bring some life to your sick and tired body.

You're straight out of the shower and over to the kettle for the first coffee of the day. While it's boiling, you throw on your work clothes and try your hardest to stop yourself looking like something from the 'night of the living dead.' The kettle boils, you pour your coffee with a few essential extra sugars this morning to really shake you into action, and you charge out of the door ready to tackle the job that you lost interest in a long time ago.

You get to work, everyone annoys you, and you keep your head down and contemplate how you're going to get through the next eight hours...

If you're smiling whilst you read this because it either describes your normal routine or at some stage in your life you've been like this or you know someone like this, then please read on...

Let me tell you something, it doesn't have to be this way. Your "Normal" routine is not how you should "Naturally" live!

Modern life can be pretty tough, everything HAS to be done immediately. We have a million ways of contacting each other and yet the art of real communication has been lost, and with the advances in technology and the growth of social media, everyone now knows your every move. This is exhausting and a lot of people are pretty sick and tired out there.

If you want to rapidly transform your body, then you need to get to know it a bit better. If you don't get this part right, none of the other bits will work!

Exhaustion, depression and a feeling of being over-whelmed are not normal behaviours. Aching muscles and constant joint pain is not something that you should just get used to, and constant tiredness, headaches and poor digestion should not be managed with stimulants and pharmaceutical drugs.

Modern science is truly amazing. We can get new functioning limbs, organ transplants, eye transplants and even hair transplants…but you know what? Your body would work really well if you just decided to look after it!

It should be the goal of everyone reading this book to get the most out of life. Generally, the only thing that prevents us achieving this goal is ourselves—the story we tell ourselves (our thoughts) and the way in which we live out our lives (our actions).

This chapter will outline the small but significant changes that you can now decide to make that will allow for rapid transformation and for you to live out the life you deserve.

I. THE PLAN

The key to creating change is to first of all understand how things are currently working. Understand that you are a very unique individual and so the way you work is going to be very different to your friend or partner. Just as we all look different on the outside, we all work very differently on the inside. That's why there is no perfect training programme or ideal diet for everyone.

There is however, a perfect way of doing things for you, you just need to understand what that is.

In order to bring about change, we first need to look at what is preventing you from achieving the body of your dreams?

In my experience, the biggest factor is stress. Whilst we all need some stress in our lives, we need deadlines, drive and determination, but we also need to know when to switch off and how to do this.

Here's the science.

Within our Central Nervous System (CNS) we have the sympathetic system – which is often known as the fight-or-flight response and activates as a result of stress placed upon it, and we have the Parasympathetic system or the rest-and-digest system – which kicks in to bring the body back to balance.

When you are in a stressed state, your breathing will alter from the effective diaphragmatic breathing pattern to shallow and anxious chest breathing. You will hold more tension in your muscles, reducing your flexibility and strength. You will also hold on to more fat, have lower energy levels and suppress your immune system.

Your body is an incredible machine and it can take pretty much anything you throw at it to survive, but this programme isn't about surviving life, it's about really thriving and that's why it's so important to address this.

We all know deep down how we feel. A number of us really do enjoy stressful situations, we love being full on or addicted to the buzz, which is fine – we need excitement in our lives. The purpose of this chapter is to encourage you to become more in touch with your body, recognise when you're really switched on and learn how to bring everything back into balance.

So how do we reduce our stress levels and achieve the body we desire?

Here's my five-step plan to bring your body back into balance, understand how it works and achieve rapid body transformation.

Step One: Sleep

You sleep when you're dead, right?! Functioning on four hours sleep is like a badge of honour to be paraded around and proudly shoved into the weaker work colleagues faces!

Well no. There's 24 hours in a day and if you're smart, you'll work for eight, rest for eight and play for eight.

This is the biggest cause of stressed, ill and dysfunctional people. If we don't allow our bodies enough time to rest and recover we will never function at an optimal level.

A lack of sleep makes you slower, depressed and more prone to illness. You can kid yourself that you can survive on four hours and it may be true, in the same way you can also survive on McDonalds for breakfast, lunch and dinner, but your body won't thank you for it!

How do you guarantee the perfect night's sleep?

Brain dump early – before you leave the office or on the commute home, make a list of all the important things you need to do the next day. Once the list is written, leave it alone. Switch off, build on your relationships outside of work and get to know the real you.

Avoid coffee after 2pm. Caffeine is a stimulant, it's the most addictive drug in the world, one cup of coffee stays in your system for up to six hours. If you drink coffee too late in the day how do you expect to switch off at night?

Make your bed a comfortable environment free from light, noise and electronic gadgets.

Buy an eye mask and drastically improve your sleep, you may look ridiculous, but who's going to see you?!

Step Two: Eat Right

The old saying "you are what you eat" is so true. You put rubbish in and you will get rubbish out. The human body is so incredible that by the time you finish reading this sentence, fifty million of your cells will have died and been replaced by others! Your liver replaces itself every five months, your lungs will renew around every two to three weeks and your taste buds will renew roughly every 10 days.

Your cells can only be as good as the fuel you provide your body with to create them. Just think about this each time you eat!

Live by these rules:

- If it's lived or comes out of the ground, eat it.

- If it comes out of a tin, a packet or a brightly coloured wrapper, don't eat it that often.

- When you go to the supermarket, just shop around the perimeter where you'll find all the good stuff, the fruit, veg, meats and fresh produce.

Step Three: Move more

A number of the other chapters are going to cover this in great detail, but know that if everyone in this world moved a bit more they would be a lot healthier, a lot happier and in a lot less pain.

Step Four: Smile

We discussed the fact that rapid body transformation starts from within. You need to change the way you act and the way that you think, and negative thoughts are a killer to any programme of change. Try to think negatively with a smile on your face...it's not going to happen.

Look for the good in others and for the fun in every element of your life and you'll go far. A number of us can too easily be accused of taking ourselves and our lives too seriously. Why do this?

Just putting a fake smile on won't cut it, you need to learn to like yourself.

The major reason people get into a bad place is because they just don't like themselves that much. If you're on your own in a room with no music, no TV and no mobile phone are you happy? If you can't be happy in your own company, how do you expect others to enjoy being around you?!

Most people avoid being on their own. They need TV and music to drown out their thoughts, they need their mobile phone like a security blanket and they require food and drink to comfort them. Don't just get to like yourself, but fall in love with yourself and really go to work on making yourself better each day. That will make you smile!

Step Five: Plan

Failing to plan is planning to fail. That may be really cheesy but it's so true. Your goal in purchasing this book is to bring about rapid change and that isn't going to happen by chance.

You need a plan to get you there – which I will provide. You just need to take the steps to make it as easy as possible to follow. Find the time to make those small changes that will make the big differences, know that it will get tough at times and have the courage to stick to it.

If you're anything like me, then you probably enjoy new challenges, new ideas and the freedom to explore them. This is great and you have to follow your passions – just know that everything works better with a bit of structure.

Plan your days, your meals, your training times and your bed times and make them happen. It's not being boring, it's living with a purpose and a structure to allow amazing things to happen.

If you want the dream body, then plan the time to get it!

Step Six: Help others

This programme is about you, so what does helping others have to do with this?

This programme is about feeling really good about yourself and nothing makes you feel good about yourself more than when you help others. As novel as its sounds, it has been scientifically proven that the secret to gain real happiness for yourself is to give to others.

It becomes infectious – if you take your mother out for lunch it makes her happy, you feel great for doing it and you're more likely to keep giving more.

This is often seen in very successful entrepreneurs who have been incredibly focussed, driven, and in most cases very selfish individuals in their pursuit of success, but when they "Get There," they realise that the extra zero's on the end of their bank accounts and the sports cars in their triple garage don't actually make them that happy, but the act of philanthropy has a strangely alluring quality.

Give more to get more, your body will thank you for it!

II. PUTTING IT IN TO ACTION

Your Morning Programme

Do This	Wake up after 8 hours of undisturbed sleep.
Why	Your body can only change when it is fully rested and recovered.
Drink This	One pint of water.
Why	It's important to hydrate first thing.
Do This	Eat Breakfast EVERY day.
Why	If you run out the door without eating breakfast, you're not only sabotaging your day but your entire training programme.
Eat This	Have protein with each meal.
Why	It's the building blocks for muscle and an appetite suppressant. Great sources for breakfast are eggs, nuts, seeds, peanut butter and meat.
Drink This	One cup of Coffee.
Why	Coffee has antioxidants that boost immunity and prevent disease. It will also provide energy and boost your metabolism.

Do This	Exercise.
Why	Starting your day with exercise to feel good, give you focus for the day and ensure that it gets done. There are too many reasons to not exercise later.
Do This	Plan your day.
Why	Write down the top three things you want to achieve today and make them happen.
Do This	Smile at someone on your way to work.
Why	Making others happy makes you happy.
Do This	Take 10 deep breaths before you start your working day.
Why	If your commute to work or any of your colleagues cause you stress learn to shut this out and start the day in a more relaxed state.

Your Afternoon Programme

Do This	Eat Lunch.
Why	It's not big or clever to work through lunch, we're building a high performance machine and that needs good quality fuel!
Do This	Laugh.
Why	Don't take yourself too seriously, have fun in everything that you do.
Stop This	Don't drink Coffee after 2 pm.
Why	Don't be an addict and don't sabotage your sleep routine! Sip water regularly throughout the day instead.
Do This	Go for a walk.
Why	Sitting at a desk all day is a sure-fire way to bring on back pain, check your posture, relax your mind and you'll be more productive as a result.

Do This	Enjoy your work.
Why	Do what you love and love what you do. You spend a third of your week working; doesn't it make sense to find something that makes you happy?

Your Evening Programme

Do This	Eat Dinner.
Why	You know this is important! Eat amazing nutritious foods and be adventurous with new recipes.
Do This	Switch off at the end of the day.
Why	Even the President has to switch off sometime. No matter how important you may think you are, the world WILL survive if you switch off your laptop!
Do This	Brain Dump.
Why	Get all of your work thoughts out and then enjoy being the real you. DON'T have a notebook by your bed; this will definitely keep you up at night.
Do This	Lights out.
Why	Create an environment for relaxation and sleep. That means no lights, no phone, no TV and no electronic devices.
Do This	Slow your breathing.
Why	Deep breathing techniques or meditation will allow your body to really switch off and you'll find it easy to fall asleep.

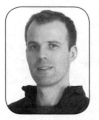

About David

David Osgathorp, BSc (Hons.) is the owner of Performance & Wellbeing Centre.

David writes:

Thanks for taking the time to find out more about me! After reading my chapter, I hope you can see how passionate I am about health and wellbeing. My goal is to make a positive impact on the lives of all my clients. I have been at the forefront of the UK Health and Fitness Industry for over ten years, and hold qualifications from some of the most prestigious personal training, sports medicine and therapy academies around the world.

As well as writing about health and wellbeing, I also walk the walk in the real world having established my own Performance & Wellbeing Centre in Highgate Village in 2006. I now have over 20 trainers, therapists and class instructors working from my 4000 square foot site in one of the most exclusive areas in London.

My multi-disciplinary approach has attracted clients from all walks of life – including athletes, actors, medical professionals and those with disabilities. I write regularly for my own in-house publications as well as for the local press, and deliver corporate wellness programmes to Fortune 500 companies on health and wellbeing in the workplace.

Enough about me, let's talk about you…

If you would like to get in touch with me please visit my website: www.davidosgathorp.com or check out my business: www.aayou.co.uk

Hope to hear from you!

David

CHAPTER 12

LAYING THE FOUNDATION FOR TRANSFORMATION SUCCESS

BY LUKA HOCEVAR

Applying training and nutrition into your lifestyle can change your health, the way your body looks, feels and performs. I think we can all agree on that.

Even though I have certain beliefs when it comes to training and nutrition, I will say that there are many programs that can get you to your goal as long as they follow certain principles.

I love writing programs and guiding clients with nutritional coaching, but the truth is that for someone to be able to follow anything with success the journey starts somewhere else. It starts in the muscle that lies in between the ears. The brain.

Working with thousands of clients in the past decade, I have realized that even when we create the best possible training and nutrition program, the client still may not follow it or do it the way they were "supposed" to. So there is something else stopping them from taking action.

My goal is to help you outline some strategies that will help you before you get started with a training and nutrition program – some strategies

119

which will help you stick with it and make progress on it, as well as conquer plateaus. Feel free to use the strategies in any area of your life you wish to improve.

Many of these strategies are based on research and real world application of brain science, psychology and behavioral change from experts in their respective fields. We have applied these same strategies into our programs at Vigor Ground and experienced some incredible changes with our clients.

When science and real world results come together, I pay attention and apply it.

Here are the three strategies that will help you…

1. FINDING YOUR "IT"

What is the one thing calling you to action right now? All of us have that one thing that drives us, the motivation to get out of bed in the morning. Maybe it's a number of things but chances are they are connected to one driving force that calls you to make the changes in your life and take action.

Most people never looked deep enough to find it so when they embark on a journey and it gets tough, they quit because the internal fire wasn't strong enough.

So what is it? What is your "IT"?

I'm talking about the deep purpose of why you decide to change. Don't think of IT as a goal, think of it as a mantra – a statement that says who you are, what drives you, and where you want to be.

It can be as little as five words, and yet, *this statement will guide your every decision and action throughout the course of the days, weeks and months of whatever transformation you choose to take on* (it will help change your behaviors).

A question I ask all my clients: "Do your behaviors match your goals?" Finding your motivation makes it more powerful because it is what influences the behaviors that then help you achieve your goals.

There is no rule for your statement. It can revolve around family, health, career, relationship, etc. as long as you dig deep enough to get to the core of what is most important to you. Once you have created the IT statement you will keep it in front of you and repeat it throughout the day. Keep it in your wallet, create a wristband out of it or have it on your screensaver. Visualize the benefits of living your life through your statement.

This statement is so important because our minds operate in three ways: the conscious, the subconscious, and the creative non-conscious process. This is how we create a vision of ourselves, which then dictates our realities. If we see ourselves in a negative light, then our subconscious will take care of it that our actions are in line with the image that we have of ourselves. A positive view translates into positive actions and the other way around.

Decisions are a result of the repetition of positive actions and thoughts. I can't emphasize enough that for success in almost anything, you need to find an inner driving force that goes beyond a training or nutrition program. You're always fueled by deeper reasons, whether you recognize it or not, so saying you just want to lose 20 lbs. is not enough. Tap into that inner drive and align it with your behaviors and actions.

Below we'll do an exercise to help you establish your IT statement.

(i). **Write down eight (8) words that are meaningful to you. Then circle the three (3) that are most important and meaningful to you right now (you can pick from some of the words in the box below*).**

(ii). **From the three words you have picked, write a story about living your best and grandest life possible and create a statement out of it.**

(iii). **Take #(ii) and cut it down to one IT statement.**

Physical Performance: Personal Best, Fitness, Power, Strength, Speed, Resilience

Pain: Function, Prevention, Movement, Freedom, Activity, Tolerance

Appearance: Comfort, Lean, Attractive, Youthful, Tone, Confident

Health: Longevity, Vitality, Spirituality, Feel Alive, Radiance, Quality of Life

Relationships: Commitment, Family, Responsibility, Connection, Presence

Energy: Empowerment, Focus, Alert, Unstoppable, Enthusiasm, Energy

Challenge: Accomplish, Exciting, Try, Goal, Evolve, Conquer

Work Performance: Creativity, Effective, Efficient, Focused, Productive, Organized

*these are some examples, feel free to add whatever you feel.

So if I picked ten words, and out of those ten the most important three for me were:

Personal Best. Family. Freedom.

My statement may be: "I will bring my Personal Best every day so that I can build a legacy through my passion and provide Freedom for my Family and myself."

My IT statement would be: "Bring Your Personal Best To Build Your Legacy And Family Freedom."

This is what matters the most to you, it fires you up and it's what you will use to keep that fire burning daily.

Now we found the fire deep inside, let's go to the next step.

2. SETTING GOALS THE *RIGHT* WAY

What are your goals? In how much detail can you answer what you are working on achieving?

"I want to get fit."

"I want to lose weight."

"I want to be leaner."

Most people are not very specific with their goals but rather general. It's a start yes, but why get "kinda" prepared for success when you can be very prepared by defining your goals very specifically?

Imagine the captain of a ship saying: "Go South!" The ship might be headed in the right general direction, but without a specific destination, it would probably get lost at sea. Do you feel you have been lost at sea when it comes to reaching your goals?

If that is the case or you are ready to make changes in any area of your life, then use this powerful ten point goal-achieving formula to get clarity on what you want in life and the mindset to be able to achieve those goals.

#1. Set Specific Goals.
The subconscious likes specific goals and the more specific they are, the easier it is to reach your goals. If you put California into the GPS it can take you many places that are very far apart and not exactly where you want to go; but if you put in the street address, city, etc. then it will get you exactly to your destination. Be specific with your goals and you will achieve specific results.

#2. Set Goals You Can Measure
You must have a way to objectively measure progress. The mirror is a great tool and one we strongly encourage (e.g., taking pictures), because ultimately the only thing that matters is that

you're happy with the way you look and feel. I will say that we perceive changes subjectively, so it's important to always have other markers too, whether weight, measurements, body fat percentage, even performance markers.

#3. Set BIG Goals.

So often people shortchange themselves and make statements like "I could never look like that" or "I'm too old." Other people buy into lower expectations of well meaning family or friends who tell them to "be realistic!" Most people get scared when setting goals and ask only for what they think they can get, NOT what they really want. This is a mistake because small goals are not motivating. Wants and big goals are!

It's okay if your goal scares you a little. Matter a fact, if your goal is not scary and exciting at the same time, then you've set too small of a goal.

#4. Set Realistic Deadlines.

How often do you see "Lose 30 lbs. in 30 days!" "Lose 10 lbs. in a weekend!" on the TV or in a magazine? Quite often I'm sure, and it's enticing, but is it possible? In some cases yes, but it's not the weight you keep off. We assess everything based on the individual. Losing 1-3 lbs. a week is a great goal.

#5. Set Long Term and Short Term Goals.

You goals list should include:

- Long term goals and your "ultimate body"

- One year goals

- Three month goals

- Weekly goals (weigh-ins, performance tests)

- Daily goals (habits to develop, behaviors to do every day)

- The goal to continuously do your best and break PR's (personal records)

Extra tip: Keep goal cards with you so you are constantly reminded of your goals. I recommend this; I have a laminated picture of my loved ones (what is important to you?) with my goals written on it in my wallet; it keeps me emotionally motivated.

#6. Focus And Prioritize On Your Main Goal

"I'd like to lose fat, gain 20 lbs. of muscle, increase speed, strength and get ready for my marathon." A goal like that is focusing on too many things and you most likely won't achieve any of them. There's a saying: "He who chases two rabbits catches neither."

Choose the most important goal to you and focus on that while giving it all your energy.

#7. WHY Do You Want To Achieve Your Goals? Attach Emotional Reasons to Your Goals.

When you discover the reason why you want to achieve your goals it adds emotional connection to it and with that, more power. The more emotion the goal generates, the more motivated you'll be to get after the goals you've set out for yourself – as well as pushing through the tough days and the hard times (and they will come).

Here are some questions that will help you determine the deep reasons for your goals?

– What's important to you about reaching your goal?

– Why is that important to you?

– How will achieving this goal impact your life? After you achieve this goal, how will you be different?

Discover the deep reasons behind your goals. This is one of the most important steps.

#8. Write Out A Goal List In The Form Of Affirmations.

The next step is to write your goal in the form of positive statements called "affirmations."

There are 3 things that will make your affirmations more powerful:

– Make personal affirmations using "I" with a verb after it. For instance "I am so happy and thankful now that I am _____ "(fill in your goal). Or, " I wake up early and take action on my goals because that is what successful people do."

– Write your affirmations in the present tense. Write, think, and visualize your goals as if you've already achieved them. Your subconscious mind works best this way.

– State your goal in positive terms. Don't say "I want to lose 40 lbs.," but rather, "I'm 40 lbs. lighter and weigh 170 lbs. at 10% body fat."

#9. Always Keep Your Goals In Front Of You So They Stay On Your Mind.

We want to embed the goals in our subconscious mind and the best way to do that is by repetition. Read your goals when you get up in the morning and before you go to bed at night and keep them in front of you throughout the day. Like I mentioned earlier, keeping then in your wallet is a great way to keep them on your mind, as is having them on your computer screen saver or on your fridge. Where do you spend the most time? Set them up there.

#10. Mentally Visualize Affirmations As If They Are Already Achieved.

Visualization means creating mental pictures or movies inside your mind; it's thinking without words. If I ask you about your ultimate body, you don't see letters spelled out bur rather a picture of that body. Your brain thinks in images. Create focused and vibrant pictures of the goals you want to achieve in your mind and they will get embedded in your mind faster and deeper than if you just write them out and read them.

We're on a roll. What now?

3. GAIN CLARITY ON WHAT TO DO NEXT

You've found your mantra.

You've gone through the goal setting process.

Now it's time to become aware of what needs to happen. Remember, awareness precedes change!

The simplest way to do this is a strategy called sentence stemming. You ask yourself a question based on your goal to find out what you need to do. You hold the answers and don't need an expert to tell you what you already know if you just ask yourself the right questions. When you do, write answers for 2-3 minutes without over-thinking, just write.

"What is important for me to do to reach _____ (your goals)?"

So, for instance: "To drop 20 lbs. I need to _____?"

If you start answering and writing things down, the answers may be something like:

- "I need to join a gym and have a structured program."

- "I need to cut down on eating fast foods and eat foods that align with my goals."

- "I need do start doing cardio several times a week."

- "I need to journal what I eat."

You will come up with whatever answers you feel will get you to your goal. Start by taking the two actions that you feel will be most important to you and sentence stem them again.

For example: "To join a gym and have a structured program, I must _____?"

The answers may be:

"—find gyms that are closest to me and fit my schedule and goals."

"—buy a book with a structured training program or look into hiring a personal trainer."

You can continue to do this with any answer and get to the exact steps you need to take to achieve success. You hold the answers.

Based on the answers, create a plan and add only as many action steps as you can handle at first. Then build on it (there are plenty of good plans in this book).

You have laid the foundation for success, keep inching away and taking action and you will achieve all the goals you set out for yourself.

I believe in you!

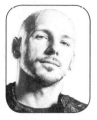

About Luka

Luka is an entrepreneur, author, strength/fitness/business coach (yes, all that), world traveler, life enjoyer (is that even a word?) and former pro-basketball player who is working on hooping consistently again. There's a lot more to him, but he'll tell you those stories over a drink some time (or maybe you can read about them on his blog).

Since he was wee little kid, Luka was entrepreneurial Unfortunately, many times it took him down the wrong path. Sports and fitness saved him. That is why these days he is all about running his businesses that are his purpose – his gym Vigor Ground Fitness and Performance which is located in Seattle, WA, and the gym he started in Slovenia, Vigor Move & Live. To serve his clients and change their lives is the internal alarm clock that gets him up in the morning.

Luka also co-wrote the national best seller, *The Fit Formula* and self-published *The Fitness Business Mixtape*. He has also written for a number of top fitness and lifestyle blogs. More than anything, he loves writing to get all the things in his head out on paper and help people find solutions (or maybe help tip them out of ambivalence on a certain matter).

Sport and fitness saved Luka's life. He was a knucklehead when he was younger. His coaches, team, family and drive to be the best basketball player (and the most capable athlete) is what tipped the scales and made him turn down a different path.

When he was done with playing professional basketball, he went into fitness (he was actually in it all that time, but that's a story for another day) and for the last decade he has been purposeful about helping people change their life through the vehicle that changed his.

Luka trains athletes, youth, and anyone that has a goal and desire to change for the better (those who don't; he helps them find it!).

To find out more about Luka, go to: www.VigorGroundFitness.com or: www.LukaHocevar.com

CHAPTER 13

THE MINIMALIST GUIDE TO GETTING RESULTS AND FINDING HAPPINESS

BY STEVE KREBS

Life is too complicated as it is, so why do we continue to make achieving the body and life of our dreams more difficult than it needs to be?

Unfortunately we live in a society of instant gratification, so many of us struggle achieving our goals. Its the "what I want vs. what I want right now" debate.

The fact of the matter is that achieving your dream body and life is not that difficult once you remove your biggest roadblock – You! Its time to get out of your own way so you can realize true happiness, health and the body you have always dreamed of. You cannot achieve a Rapid Body Makeover without first Making Over your Mind, habits and actions first.

So here we go!

THE CHALLENGE:

It takes around 30 days to develop a lasting behavior change.

1. Select one habit you want to eradicate, and the habit you will replace it with.

2. Have a plan. Be very specific and put together your plan of action for the 30 days. Make sure that you have a support and accountability system in place, who will you report to? Finding a buddy to participate with you will be super helpful.

3. Make it public. Let everyone know what you are going to do. Post it on Facebook (during one of your scheduled FB times) and let the world know your intentions and commitment.

4. Let them know. Let your support and accountability group know what you are up to.

5. "It's a CELEBRATION!" <insert Rick James voice here> After the 30 days, reward yourself for the HUUUGE shift you have made in your life and don't look back!

This works time and time again because of a few factors:

- Commitment

- Accountability

- Encouragement

- Inspiration

Our habits are what decide our direction in life. They directly affect our happiness, finances, health, relationships.... okay, they affect our entire lives. So please do not take them lightly and realize that you have 100% control of your habits, and therefore your life.

"Small daily improvements over time lead to stunning results."

YOUR MISSION:

Rick Hansen, the man who traveled around the world in his wheelchair was asked the "secret" of achieving this exceptional feat. He said that rather than focusing on the 24,901 miles he had to cover, he simply thought only about one session at a time, 23 miles per session, 3 sessions per day.

Rick Hansen is living proof that you can accomplish anything if you fully commit to it, put a plan together and follow the damn plan.

He started off small. His small victories lead him to large ones.

"Thinking always ahead, thinking always of trying to do more, brings a state of mind in which nothing is impossible."

Your thoughts are living things that direct your actions each day. If you fill your mind with goals, possibilities and positivity, you will follow the same path as Rick Hansen. You will achieve things you never thought possible, and live a life of purpose, passion and accomplishment.

You control your thoughts.

You control your actions.

Stop giving up control of your life by living reactively. Take full responsibility for your place in life. Take action on the things that you are in control of -- like your thoughts, actions, exercise, nutrition, environment and education.

Sometimes we struggle in life because we don't have a "compass" to guide us towards the right path. If you don't know where you are going, then it's pretty damn difficult to get there.

So lets figure out what you stand for. Your homework for today is to write out your *Personal Mission Statement for Life*. This will be your "guiding light" or GPS system, a clear statement of where you are going in life.

To help you out, here is my personal mission statement for life:

"My mission in this life is to be the happiest, most giving and caring person I know. I will live with loyalty, honor and respect. I will provide for my family financially and with love and support. I will leave my footprint on this world."

Put your mission statement where you can see it everyday, like on your bathroom mirror. Read this mission statement a MINIMUM of twice daily. Make it a part of your early morning ritual of improvement.

If a man can wheelchair around the world, just imagine what you are capable of.

THE PROMISE:

When you make a promise do you always follow through?

"A promise means everything. But once it is broken, sorry means Nothing."

Life goes by so fast, and we all get caught up in the "rat race", but being busy is NOT an excuse for missing out on the important things in life. So much of our time is spent on things that don't matter... Television, Facebook, Video Games, Drama, negative people, bad relationships, addictions, etc., etc.

We are all guilty of breaking promises. We have all let down people we love, but that doesn't mean we can't make a promise to ourselves that we won't tolerate that behavior from this point forward.

To change your outer world, you must first change your inner world.

People who break promises to their loved ones are usually notorious for breaking the promises they make to themselves as well. It starts from the inside, and works its way out.

Homework for today: Write out any and all promises you have broken to yourself. Remember that AWARENESS PRECEDES CHANGE. You have to bring these past let-downs into the light, so that we can learn from them, and move forward.

Its time to follow through on ALL of your promises, because if you don't what's the point of making them in the first place? You are worth it.

Remember that the only proof of living is growth, and the only guarantee in life is change. Don't fight it, embrace it.

Make the decision to be the best version of you each day.

REMOVE OBSTACLES:

(i). Stop Worrying:

> *"I've had a lot of trouble in my life, some of which*
> *actually happened."*
> ~ Mark Twain

Too many people are spending the best years of their lives stuck in a constant state of worry. The unfortunate thing is that the majority of the worries are concocted in our own minds. These negative thoughts are slowly "cooked" until they grow exponentially and become a Monster in our minds.

So many of the things I worried about, or dwelled on ended up never happening or happened, but were nowhere near as severe as I made them out to be in my mind.

What we focus on grows. So if you continue to focus on what you don't have, or what might happen, you will increase the occurrence of anxiety, worry, depression and unhappiness. You will cement the feeling of discontent.

Most worry and anxiety stems from lack of control. Most of the problems we think are disasters turn out to be blessings, in hindsight.

The fact of the matter is, most of the things we worry about can actually help us grow. If we CHOOSE to see these challenges for what they are, a chance for us to grow and improve, then the anxiety and worry will subside.

There is, in the worst fortune, the best chances for a happy change.

Homework: List out all the things that worry you. Put Stars next to anything that you worry about daily. Then next to the worry write out the worst thing that can happen, and then write out what you can learn from this. Take the power away from the worry, focus on the solution and what you can learn from it.

(ii). Stop Rushing:

"Nature does not hurry, yet everything is accomplished."
~ Lao Tzu

That quote honestly changed my life. I was the guy who constantly felt the need to be busy. Notice I didn't say productive.....

Our society has turned into one gigantic hamster wheel. Round and round we go.

We have more ways to stay in contact then ever before, but our relationships have suffered. We have more weight-loss solutions but more obesity. We have more stuff, but less happiness. We fill our days with the things we think we "should" be doing, instead of just slowing life down and enjoying the path.

Constantly being in a hurry just reveals how inept we are at time management, organization and planning. Not having enough time is the #1 excuse on the planet. It is applied to everything from why you didn't follow through with your nutrition, or why you missed a workout, to why you didn't show up for a loved one, etc., etc., etc.

We all have the same 24 hours in a day. How is that successful people get so much done in a short amount of time? It's all about organization and time mastery. Remember that "Time Mastery is Life Mastery."

So before you start saying that you are different, and you HAVE to hurry because you have no time, just read this:

If you sleep seven hours a night and work eight hours a day you still have sixty-three hours of free time every week! This amounts to 252 hours every month and 3,024 hours every single year.

Simplifying your life and becoming more productive are actually quite simple. All you have to do is develop the HABIT. Daily habits are what will ultimately decide the direction of your life. You may "already know" what you need to do, but you have to actually take action on it to elicit a positive response. *[Remember that the words "I Already Know That." are the most dangerous words in the English Language].*

Feeling overwhelmed causes anxiety and stress. Anxiety and stress will cause you to freeze. Once you freeze your life is on pause. It's time to put together a plan of action, reset the program in your brain, and start living life with purpose and passion.

STAY MOTIVATED:

Here are 20 ways to keep yourself motivated:

1: Don't bite off more than you can chew. When setting a new goal like losing body fat, most people come out like gangbusters. They try to make enormous changes, and then fail when they don't see the results they are looking for within a few days.

2: Just get your ass moving. There are going to be days when you don't want to get out of bed to train, on those days make yourself just get your ass moving. The first step is the toughest.

3: Buddy System. Make sure you have someone to hold you accountable. Doing what you said you will do is an amazing habit to develop, having someone to make sure you do it is priceless. The buddy system works on so many different levels, and is ultimately why Next Level is so successful.

4: Eradicate Negative Thoughts. Immediately replace a negative thought with a positive one. You have about .25 seconds to replace the negativity before its too late. Practice this every day. Remember that the only way to develop a habit is to do it consistently.

5: Focus on the Prize! Stop focusing on how difficult it's going to be to make the change, and focus on how you will look and feel after it is accomplished. Remember only positive thoughts are allowed. If a man can wheelchair across the world, I think you can get your ass out of bed and exercise....

6: Get FIRED UP again. Find pictures, videos, or motivational quotes that remind you why you started this change in the first place. Look at them every morning as a part of your morning rituals.

7: Feed your brain. Read a book or story about someone who has overcome insurmountable odds to achieve success. This will add fuel to your fire.

8: Surround yourself with a support team. Find like-minded people who are driving towards the same goal. Hang more with friends who understand your change, and will never sabotage you. *Birds of a feather flock together.* :-)

9: Build on your successes. Celebrate each step along your journey and ENJOY IT. Remember the path is better than the end. Don't wish your life away. Enjoy the process of change.

10: Fight through the tough times. Everyone messes up. It's only a mistake if you repeat it. So if you "cheat" just leave it in the past, and move forward. Right the ship. Don't allow one bad decision sabotage all of your goals.

11: Ask for help. Never be too proud to seek out the help of others.

12: Track your progress. This is a simple way to maintain your motivation by consistently seeing how much progress you have made.

13: Reward yourself. If you hit a milestone, go buy yourself something nice. My advice is to never reward yourself with food though. You are not a dog, don't exacerbate the problem.

14: Set benchmarks. These are smaller steps you can take that are guaranteed to succeed. They help build momentum, and once you get that, you will be unstoppable.

15: Find a Teacher, Mentor or Coach. Having a coach is one of the smartest things that you can do. Everyone should have a coach.

16: Never miss 2 days in a row. Habits are easier to break than to develop. Make the commitment to never miss 2 days in a row of training, clean eating etc.

17: Visualize it. See yourself at the end of the journey looking and feeling amazing. Spend 10 minutes a day in quiet reflection focusing on this very thing. First you create it internally, then you can manifest it externally.

18: Awareness precedes change. Be aware of your urges to quit, and stop them in their tracks.

19: See the good in it. You won't stick to a change if you don't have any enjoyment in it. Focus on the pleasurable aspects of the process.

20: Be Stubborn. Don't allow the weak negative voice in your head to talk you out of what you really want. You deserve this. So fight for it!

If you want something bad enough, you will find a way to make it happen. Think about the last time you were in a store and saw something you just "had to have." I'm sure you figured out how you could get it on the spot, and you made it happen.

It just shows that in the right circumstances, you have the ability to maintain motivation, develop a plan, and execute the plan. So stop bullshitting yourself!

<u>Stop thinking its too hard to eat clean, to exercise, to achieve your goals, and just MAKE THE DECISION to keep going until you get there.</u>

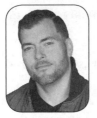

About Steve

Steve Krebs is co-founder of The Pack Fitness Business and also Changing the Game: The Fitness Business Event. Steve coaches fit pros and facility owners on how to run a high profit performance and fitness facility. Steve has been running fitness and performance facilities for 12 years, and has successfully operated Next Level Athletic Performance Inc. for eight years in an area ranked in the top ten places to own a business in Forbes Magazine. The Pack Fitness Business Mentorship is known for transforming businesses, in turn transforming the lives of its members and their families.

You can find more information on coaching at:
www.thepackfitnessbusiness.com

CHAPTER 14

MOM MATTERS TOO

BY TRICIA BURNS

Mom!? Mom, will you get me this? Mom, I need your help! Mom, I am hungry! Honey, when is dinner? Honey, we are out of groceries. Do you have the laundry done? Honey, did you get the bills paid? Mom, I need cupcakes for school tomorrow. We have company coming tomorrow, do you have the house cleaned?

If any of this sounds familiar to you, you are a busy mom like myself and approximately 85 million other American women. Taking time for ourselves becomes a rare commodity.

Before I go any further, let me tell you a story about a new mom of a little boy and four bonus children. A mom that was once told that carrying a baby would not be an option, was suddenly in the full swing mother mode! Being a rancher's wife means the work is never done, add owning/operating a nail salon with motherhood, and you have a perfect recipe for no time for yourself.

For 3 years I thought I had a great handle on being a full time mom to one, and part time mom to four, wife, and entrepreneur. A typical wife and mother with regular duties. Wake up, get ready for work, son ready for daycare, and head out the door for work. Work that seemed so fulfilling, a happy place. What is the worst thing that can go wrong in a nail salon, right? The wrong color of polish is an easy fix! I'd come home from a day of helping women feel better about themselves make dinner, clean up, do the laundry, bathe my child and put him to bed shortly before I crashed, amid pairing socks.

But, no worries, I'd think, I've got this! After all, there are moms that are A LOT busier than myself. I wouldn't complain or ask for help because this is what being a mother and wife is all about. If I didn't have a job, would others think I was lazy? If I asked for help does that mean I am not good enough? I have an idea, I will just purchase more pre-made food because that will free up some extra time preparing meals, and then I can help my hard working husband outside more. After all, he works many more hours and a much more physically demanding job than I!

Soon, the few little things I did for myself became a distant memory. Thank goodness for HIIT workouts, because I could find 15-20 minutes every other day!

Just when I thought I could not squeeze one more thing into my day, we received great news, three of my four bonus children were moving in!! What an exciting day! The moving day arrived and soon we were getting ready for two children to start high school, one in middle school, and the youngest in daycare. My days went from busy to hectic! I still felt that even though my workload had greatly increased, I should still be able to manage it all – there are mothers with far more children than four. There are women that balance far more than I do, right?

Our nutrition declined, as it was more about convenience, not health. I became more tired and soon I opted to sleep that extra half of an hour instead of getting up to work out. Days went by and the more tired I became. I thought this is just the life of a busy mom, suck it up! The downward nutritional cycle continued as we ran to activities and school events. I added my morning workouts to my list of things of the past.

What I didn't realize at the time was that everything works hand in hand. The age-old concept of cause and effect. As my nutrition deteriorated, so did my energy. I wasn't fueling my body properly. The more I omitted doing anything for MYSELF, the more I felt defeated.

Working out was not a priority because it was my job to be mom, wife, and nail salon owner/operator – other women do it without complaint, so should I!

As my family and clients saw that time for myself wasn't important to me, they felt as if they could ask for more of my time. Soon I felt I was being pulled in every direction, and it was because of the example I set. The standard I had put in place about how to treat me!

As the result of many positive changes in my life I now know two thing:

• If you don't take care of yourself, nobody else will.

• If you are not healthy, neither is your family!

I am now a personal fitness trainer, wellness coach, and lifestyle weight management specialist. I am so excited to share with you five easy steps on how to get you and your family healthy!

I will show you!

Through (1) goal setting, (2) nutrition, (3) strength training, (4) cardio, and (5) attitude.

You can feel so different in Only 21 Days!

GOAL SETTING IS THE MOST IMPORTANT FACTOR IN CHANGE

We can't achieve if we do not know what it is we want, plain and simple! Set a date or specific details for the end result. That's just the way we operate! If you were given an assignment in school with no end date, chances are you would never complete it!

Goals need to be specific, so you'll know which part of the process you're in and the ways in which you will achieve it. You have to have a plan!

Most people have goals to get in shape, lose weight, fit into my "skinny" clothes, etc., but these are vague and your mind becomes confused about what's truly meant. General descriptions do not have boundaries, so you always leave room for mistakes and compromise. If you want results that you can be proud of, be specific! To be specific, include all specific details. Write down something like, "I want to weigh 120 pounds by October of this year." or "My body fat percentage will be 20% by June of this year," or "I want to lower my total cholesterol to 200." Include names, the specific number, the amount, the date and everything else needed to train your mind to work towards that goal.

We need measurable goals. You can then gauge how well you have done throughout the journey. Stop to celebrate each victory along the way Measurable details give us specifics for our success. For your health and wellness goals, include details such as specific numbers, cutting out certain foods, a set amount of time to exercise per day or week, etc. Always use measurable details so you can understand how close you are to getting to your goals. If your goal is to lose twenty pounds, then losing ten pounds is halfway. Celebrate!

Only set goals that are possible. Some people set goals too high to reach, setting themselves up for failure. This causes frustration. Always look how far you have come and not how far you have left to go! Some goals can be achieved faster compared to others if you have some strengths and paths to back these up. Use strategy for big objectives.

You won't finish anything without deadlines! Stay specific when setting timelines and schedules. For example, indicate things like "To spend an hour working out every day starting tomorrow (indicate exact date and year)." Setting the exact time and date will spur you to start working on your goals Some goals take longer to accomplish, so it's wiser to break these into smaller objectives, complete with deadlines. You can finish everything in a sequence to reach the biggest one.

PROPER NUTRITION IS VITAL!

You have heard it said a million times, "You can't outwork a poor diet."

What we use as fuel for our bodies is going to determine how efficiently our bodies work and ultimately look! Nutrition can be complex to understand! Every day we watch TV, read a magazine, or look at our computers and there is a new food that we should eat. Tomorrow it may just be the food they are now telling you NOT to eat! There are more than 73,000 published books on amazon.com about nutrition, so I am going to keep it simple...EAT CLEAN WHOLE FOODS! Cut out processed foods, sugars, "bad" carbohydrates, and GMOs (to name a few).

Last but not least, drink WATER, lots and lots of water! Bodies must have water to function!

When we cut out "toxic" foods we promote a healthy physiological and hormonal response. We support a healthy gut, immune function, and minimize inflammation. Your relationship with food and how your metabolism responds to food will shift once you cut out toxic food. You will experience more energy, better mood, improved sleep, less gastrointestinal stress, and lose weight among many other benefits. Your body will stop demonstrating symptoms of toxicity including bad breath, bloating, gas, constipation, and skin conditions. Fatigue and puffy eyes may well disappear! There are more serious conditions such as: arthritis, asthma & allergies, auto-immune diseases, chronic fatigue syndrome, diabetes, high blood pressure, high cholesterol, obesity, acne, eczema, fibromyalgia, food allergies, headaches, heart disease, irritable bowel syndrome, menopausal symptoms, and menstrual problems that can be solved by your diet.

Your body deserves to be treated as a high performing machine and must be fueled accordingly!

NOW LET'S TALK ABOUT EXERCISE!

Cardio was the "must do" exercise in the late 80's and 90's, but since then new research has emerged. Steady state cardio has been found to not be as effective as once thought.* It was in the late 90's that a Japanese researcher discovered the benefits of a high intensity interval

(HIIT) cardio training was far superior to steady state cardio. HIIT includes short bursts of high intensity cardio followed by short periods of active rest. HIIT training also improves muscle endurance and actual fat loss.

A HIIT workout is the most effective and beneficial to your body when performed every other day.

Strength training is also a must when transforming your body. Let me start out by making it very clear that proper strength training will NOT bulk you up! That is a huge misconception. Muscle is the only true fountain of youth and any age or gender can start strength training! What strength training will do is tone your body, make your body lean, utilize the energy properly and not store it as FAT! Changing your body composition will not only increase your energy but also your self-confidence, self-worth, and your self-esteem. Did you know when you are sleeping, your muscles burn 25% of your energy or calories? So, the more muscle, the more calories burned, even while you are sleeping!!

Well-conditioned muscles are vital in performing everyday tasks without the risk of injury! Our muscles are shock absorbers and also balancing agents. Having an effective strength training work out does not have to include expensive equipment, dumbbells, or a gym membership. Using body weight and traditional strength training (i.e., lunges, squats, push-ups, wall sits) will get you the same results!

Attitude: For your rapid body transformation you need the right attitude! A positive attitude makes us happier, but did you know it makes you healthier too! You are the head coach of your thoughts and your thoughts all play on the team of attitude!

IN SUMMARY

These steps will change your body, your life, and the health and happiness of your family. It's fail proof! Write down your goals. Once you have done this you can use the other four components; nutrition, cardio, strength training, and attitude to construct your road map.

Start your journey today! Begin enjoying the results of your body transformation!

*According to a 2011 study in the scientific journal, *Psychoneuroendocrinology*, cardio increases the stress hormone cortisol. (Skoluda, N., Dettenborn, L., et al. Elevated Hair Cortisol Concentrations in Endurance Athletes. *Psychoneuroendocrinology*. September 2011) Performing steady state cardio puts massive amounts of stress on your body and increases your cortisol hormone.

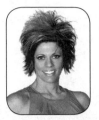

About Tricia

'My passion is helping others achieve their goals! The reward is when a client gains control of their destiny by becoming healthy! I feel blessed to be able to help my clients. I look forward to helping you too!'

~ Tricia B, Co-Author

Tricia's son's birth 6½ years ago was the trigger for her fitness. Like many others, Tricia wanted to get into pre-baby clothes. She leads a busy life – five children, husband and a ranch! Her wonderful husband Marty, a weightlifter, suggested she start working out. It was at that point she found her passion!

Between the ranch, her salon and her family - time was scarce. Although enjoyable, she was soon discussing nutrition and fitness more than nails!

She took an enviable leap of faith and followed her dream! She completed her Personal Fitness Trainer as well as the Lifestyle Weight Management Specialist courses and, believing that fitness starts inside, trained as a Wellness Coach. She is a vibrant motivational speaker. Experienced with clients of all ages, she assists clients define their goals and regain confidence. Her popularity is widespread.

"I want you to know about the personal attention you will receive. In me, you will discover an honest, hard -working coach! As a fitness professional, these qualities are vital. I will demonstrate a high standard of professionalism and confidentiality." ~ Tricia B. Co-Author

Explore your potential with her principles of **Inspiration, Fitness and Nutrition.**

For questions, information, press enquiries:

tricia@team-burns.com

Your transformation is about to start!

CHAPTER 15

STRESS EXERCISE LOVE FOOD

THE RECIPE FOR RAPID BODY MAKEOVERS – YOUR RELATIONSHIP WITH SELF

BY KESSEA MOSES

As an entrepreneur starting a vastly growing company…

A casualty of several unsuccessful relationships…

A Midwest native that loves *hotdish*…

It shouldn't be any surprise that one day I woke up, looked in the mirror, and asked myself,

"When did this happen?"

It's true, that morning started out like any other. I jumped out of bed. Made sure the kids got to school. I fed the dog but there wasn't time for a walk. I rushed through my shower, picked out my clothes, and then it happened; I caught a very awkward view of my backside in the mirror and knew, life as I had known it had to change.

Change, that six-letter word that often stands between us and what we want to achieve. Once we recognize "change", the next step should be easy; we plot out a course to get us there. In my case, the destination

149

was half my body size. So I sat down with my pad of paper, turned on my inner businesswoman, and went to work to create this road map for body transformation.

I remember thinking. I lost almost 100 pounds twice before, what helped me back then? Could I do enough exercise with the schedule I held and the physical limitations I had? And I remember fearing; I feared the amount of time the weight had been on my body, along with my age, was now working against me.

I tried several low calorie diets. I even lost a few pounds but quickly gained them back along with several more once I discontinued their program. I found a life coach. I read articles relating weight to hidden obstacles and I knew, I had obstacles! However, when I was spending time being coached, I didn't have time for exercise so I made the choice to hit the gym full speed ahead instead.

What did I learn? I had it all backwards. More is better when it comes to eating healthy foods. Less and consistent is more successful with regards to exercise, and support is not a choice. There truly is a recipe for body makeovers but it is one that most of us follow incorrectly.

Stress: is the body's natural response to change. Each of us are programmed to handle stress; this has been proven through the testing of our hormones and our body's reaction when faced with fear, excitement, challenges, and pain. In the "customary state," as the body encounters stress, the brain sends a warning through our neurotransmitters. Our organs respond by releasing chemicals such as norepinephrine and cortisol. Once the stressor is removed, the body calms the nervous and endocrine systems – bringing the body back into balance. This process is known as "the fight-or-flight response" and is vital for our survival. This is the same response that gives us the additional strength and endurance we need when faced with a stimulus. Unfortunately, stress is often undervalued as a medical condition and frequently regarded as just part of life. To fully understand the traumatic impact stress can have on the body, we must first look at what our body is intended to endure and how these hormones affect our overall health when in balance.

Cortisol plays an essential role in reaching goals related to fitness, weight, and wellness. It also plays a significant role in maintaining our body's insulin levels, blood pressure, metabolizing fat, immune function, and inflammatory response. So what happens when we overlook the balance that must be kept between our goals and the natural role of our body's systems? Our body moves towards disease, including obesity, and further away from wellness.

When stress hormones are in play, the increased level of cortisol shuts down our metabolic processes, slowing digestion, and limits our body's ability to grow and fight infection while diverting all new energy (the calories we consume) to storage vs. utilization for energy. In doing so, we prepare ourselves for the upcoming challenge. However, when challenges cease to end, much like in the state of our fast-paced lives, our body fails to stop the production of these hormones. This is also a common reaction in the world of extreme exercise and dieting.

The process for change is not one size fits all; each of us has our limit to the amount of stress we can endure. When we reach this limit, we overproduce hormones which aid in weight gain, depression, anxiety, sleeplessness, brain fog, memory impairment, digestive concerns, and heart disease. When we extreme diet and overtrain, we inadvertently put our body into a state of chronic stress. This state prevents us from efficiently burning fat – while forcing our body to turn on itself through catabolism (see segment regarding food).

Exercise: as defined: Any activity that enhances or maintains our physical fitness and overall health and wellness. So why are we focused on the extreme and less mindful of the lack of movement in our daily routines?

Let us first revisit what we just learned. When our body is under stress, our hormones prevent us from reaching our goals. Knowing this to be fact, it can be assumed that one who has never ran a mile would be putting their body at risk should they set out to run a marathon. This can also be assumed when one who has never attempted to weight train signs up for CrossFit with the belief that they will be able to keep up with the class. Fortunately, we have educated trainers that prevent this type of mishap from occurring. Unfortunately, we have trainers who are not experts in their field and an even higher number of us that feel we can't afford the investment for proper base-building training. The answer: simplify what it is you need to support your vision.

Your vision is free; it's what you picture your ultimate self to be. Exercise is merely a factor of this vision and should not be given the power of control for overall health. What does this mean? If your goal is to lose fat, exercise will play a key role in obtaining this goal. However, so will managing stress, sleep, support, and the foods you consume. The amount of fat you wish to burn, along with the physical endurance you currently have, should determine the exercise plan you choose. The good news, losing fat doesn't take much exercise. You can lose fat just by increasing your daily activity. In fact, this is the best place to start.

In my field of expertise, body makeovers, I frequently find myself encouraging clients to slow down. During my own experience with losing weight, I had to learn to slow down as well. The concept of "no pain, no gain" felt true to my core and the theory of more is better is taught throughout our society. To question these values felt controversial – yet my results stood on their own.

My results: Calories burned has limits just as calories consumed. At the start of my program, my ideal recipe for caloric burn was two days of strength training, two days of rest, and three days of 30-minute cardio bursts. When I increased my cardio to 60 minutes, my body used stored energy from my muscles vs. burning fat. Finding this magic formula was the key to my success. Why you ask?

Muscle burns far more calories than fat and the volume of fat I had was far greater than that of my muscle mass. By working out at a rate too extreme for my body, I was consistently breaking down muscle to gain access to stored energy. Once I converted and worked out at the level of intensity that kept my body within my "fat zone", I increased my aerobic threshold teaching my body to burn fat for energy while increasing my metabolism and growing muscle mass.

Love: a four-letter word. For the purpose of this chapter, I will refer to love as those that offer you support; who unconditionally care for your wellbeing and your personal growth.

Let me share a story of how I found support. It came to me at a time I reached a plateau in my weight loss and from a man I never met prior to this moment. I share this because often I hear people limiting their perceptions of support. They think of family, friends, co-workers, and possibly their children. Many of us that struggle with weight also struggle with obstacles within these same relationships; we feel alone, isolated, and may have already withdrawn. For those of you who live like I did, surrounded by people who validate your pain and offer support through reassurance, I ask that you entertain the idea that there may be another way.

After receiving the prestigious award of Office of the Year, I was asked to speak at our national convention. I was encouraged to share my challenges, my personal story, and the pain that aided me along the way. In doing so, I knew I was going to be vulnerable; vulnerable to the perceptions of those in the audience.

In preparation for this speech, I set out to lose as much weight as possible. I crash-dieted, overexercised, and looked for support in all the wrong places; I failed miserably. I failed to accept myself for the woman I was, to love myself, and to forgive myself. I failed to give myself permission to be proud of my accomplishments. I focused only on my failures, not ever hearing my strengths.

When my day came to present, I had destroyed my metabolism. The extreme training and dieting resulted in my weight plateau. Nevertheless, I followed through on my commitment and I presented my story to a group of several hundred respected colleagues; one can only imagine my cortisol level that day. The objective of my speech was to encourage others...to reach those that may feel insignificant, letting them know they aren't far off the path of us larger offices. What happened next was a lesson for me; a lesson that changed my spirit indefinitely.

The following morning, as I hid in the back of the room, I had the honor of hearing a story of how another overcame their obstacles and gain health and wellness. As this man told his story, the room drew silent. He had the attention of every person, myself included. He talked about his experiences, how he lost 164 pounds, the challenges he faced, and the perceptions of our society. When he was almost done with his story, he paused briefly then stated, "I am not hero in the room, it is people like Kessea Moses that are the real hero in my mind." This wasn't an ordinary man, this was Bill Germanakos. The winner of the 4th season of the Biggest Loser and he was sharing his stage with me; I mattered.

That was all it took for me to refocus my efforts. I mattered; I had the power to make a difference and the messages embedded in my mind could be rewritten to represent strength and empowerment.

<u>Food!!</u> By far my favorite part of body makeovers because you get to eat yourself skinny! If you do nothing else suggested in these pages, please show your body some love through eating healthy. The number one mistake I see people make is that they limit themselves to a ridiculous amount of calories. I apologize for the judgment but not the message; people need to stop encouraging starvation as a means to healthier living.

I'm typically the bearer of bad news when I say there is no magic pill and when it sounds too good to be true, it generally is. So, what does a healthy nutrition plan look like? It's different for each of us. This is why we hear stories of a plan working for one but not another.

Nutrition should encourage muscle maintenance, or muscle growth, along with fat maintenance or fat loss. When measuring success, don't rely on BMI (body mass index) as a tool for health.

BMI does not take into consideration your muscle mass resulting in athletes being considered obese, due to muscle weighing more than fat, and the new classification of "skinny fat" – when an individual has the recommended BMI but lacks the desire muscle mass for optimal health. At our center, we use InBody to measure the percent of lean mass; a noninvasive machine recently endorsed by the Biggest Loser.

When tracking changes in muscle and fat, take note of what the changes are. Typically, a decrease in muscle mass, with an increase in body fat, represents too few calories. An increase in muscle mass, with an increase in body fat, represents too many calories. A decrease in muscle mass, as well as a decrease in body fat, represents a diet low in protein. By tweaking nutrients, you'll be well on your way for your rapid body makeover.

Tweaking, not to be mistaken with twerking, involves minor adjustments to the macronutrients you consumed. I encourage real food, all food groups, and lots of it; you should eat every 3-4 hours. The amount one eats depends on the individual; the more you weigh, the higher your activity intensity, and your age all play roles in the amount of carbohydrates, proteins, and fats you should consume. I recommend working with a certified nutritionist for this step. However, if you want to get started on your own, start by avoiding refined starches and eating foods in their natural state; processed foods tend to be high in fat, sodium, or sugar.

Divide food into 5 to 6 portions; 3 meals and 2-3 snacks. Always eat a protein with a carbohydrate to help control your insulin level. Eat foods that have less than 20% of their carbohydrates coming from sugar and drink/eat half your body weight daily in fluids. Consume fiber and don't skip your meals/snacks. This means, you may need to eat a snack rich in protein after dinner if your dinner falls before 7pm. Often people refrain from eating after 6pm based on old science and teachings. This puts the body into a state of catabolism during the night.

As you sleep, your body is at work repairing the "damage" you endured during the day – restoring tissues to support the new you. This work puts much demand on your body; a mindful evening snack will keep you on track. It is equally important to never skip breakfast. As you awake, your body is in need of new energy sources. Understanding these demands may shed light on why those that eat breakfast are found to have better body fat percentages than those that don't. If you follow these steps and still struggle with fat loss, I recommend an easy blood test to check for food intolerances.

More information regarding food intolerances can be found on our website: www.mnwellnesscoaching.com.

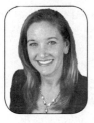

About Kessea

Kessea Moses is a Best Selling Author, a CFNS instructor, Founder and former CEO of Physicians ExamOne, President of Peace of Mind Diagnostics, and Co-Founder of Minnesota Wellness Coaching. Her expertise in Strength Rehabilitation (CSRS), Boot Camps, Wellness, and Nutrition make her one of the world's number one go-to authorities in overall health.

At the age of only 42, Kessea was presented with an opportunity to retire. After much sole searching, she made a profound decision to do the opposite; Kessea expanded her operations with the single objective to help others become a survivor vs. a victim of circumstance.

As a survivor herself, Kessea has undergone 10 knee surgeries, hip surgery, struggles with hip dysplasia, and faces dual hip and knee replacements in the years to come. At the age of 9, she overheard her doctors stating, "At the rate Kessea's knees are declining, she will be in a wheelchair by the age of 25."

At the age of 14, Kessea experienced the loss of her brother to suicide and shortly thereafter, her father was diagnosed with cancer and in need of a heart transplant. Experiences of childhood abuse lead to a diagnosis of Post Traumatic Stress Disorder and at the age of 39, she started treatment for epilepsy; Kessea understands physical and metal challenges.

The messages from "Kessea's beginning" played repeatedly in her head. She didn't feel she could keep herself safe and she felt happiness was impossible. It was at the point of hitting "bottom" that she learned she was pregnant; pregnant for the 5th time, she had already lost 4 children to miscarriages. Fortunately, this time was different, Kessea gave birth to a healthy baby girl. She also gave birth to a new life and a new body. That's right, Kessea was considered high risk, restricted, and had gained over 70 pounds.

Kessea was successful in losing her pregnancy weight – which aided in her new-found courage to question what else she could accomplish if she put her mind to it. Within the next two years, Kessea developed an idea for a company, found customers to support it, and secured an opportunity to have her idea funded by a 3rd party. In 2001, she purchased the rights to this company and since has grown it to be a multimillion-dollar organization.

Within this same time period, Kessea gave birth to another healthy baby girl, and was faced once again with the task of losing another 70 pounds. Yet, this time was different. She was also met with a slowing metabolism. Limited by western medicine, Kessea set out to learn everything she could regarding body transformation. In 2009, she reached her goal of 16 % body fat and has kept the extra weight off since.

Presently, Kessea has dedicated her career to helping others reach their wellness goals and sharing her secrets for Body Transformation. In 2013, Kessea participated in her first 5K. She placed first and second, during the same race, but that is a story for another book.

www.mnwellnesscoaching.com

CHAPTER 16

HEALTHY HABITS CREATE YOUR HEALTHY LIFE

BY ERIKA BINGER

When I was a child, I remember being so active and playing outdoors continuously without thinking, planning or considering how my body was responding to any activity. At the time, I wasn't consciously considering how what I was doing would impact my health, but it was actually laying the foundation for a life of health. I didn't know much about being healthy, watching what I ate, counting calories or staying in shape. I knew what was fun and how to keep my imagination active. My brother, sister and I would spend countless hours creating games to keep ourselves occupied. We would play outside, in the yard, climb over obstacles and trees or play in the local park. We'd play chase, freeze tag, follow-the-leader, hide-and-seek, jump rope or hopscotch. We'd play on the jungle-gym set, swing, teeter-totter and flip off the bars. We'd climb to the top of the hill, run down and do it again. If we couldn't get outdoors, many of our activities would transfer indoors: we'd play hide-and-seek, chase each other around the house, do gymnastics, sometimes jump on the bed (if mom wasn't around) and make up numerous other activities.

We weren't the only ones establishing good habits. Our father ran nearly every day and our mother walked each morning. They enjoyed playing tennis, skiing and swimming – at least Dad did, Mom would teach us! Little did we know she despised the water, but because she believed it was vitally important for us to learn to swim, she never let on. She overcame her anxiety, only revealing to us as we became more proficient in swimming and mature, her feelings towards water. Our meals were usually comprised of meat (mainly beef), some carbohydrates and always fresh vegetables, with the occasional salad and desert. Beverages would be milk and maybe water. We grew up being physically active and eating a well-balanced diet. These two components seemingly laid the foundation for a healthy life.

Similar to our upbringing, you may have also had experiences growing up when movement was easy and second nature. You may have had boundless energy when you were younger, and climbing stairs was simple. Walking around the neighborhood or chasing after a ball didn't cause your breath to shorten or your muscles to ache. You may have felt like you could play all day and never get exhausted. You were constantly on the go but never perceived it as exercise or a form of staying healthy; it just was your normal. You didn't really think too much about moving or about what you ate. You might even have been able to eat whatever you wanted, despite not being too physically active. Now, though, the pounds seem to have crept on your frame and the food you are putting into your body isn't really satisfying you much. Worse yet, it may even leave you hungry. You may find yourself settled into your career, juggling school and work, family, budgeting and not having a lot of time. Whether this resonates with you or not, some key components are central to being healthy now.

Trying to create set-aside time for yourself to work out may not seem realistic, and it shouldn't have to be separate from your everyday life and who you are. Being active and healthy is a lifestyle choice and needs to be integrated into everything you do. It should be what you enjoy and like.

Have you been trying to get healthier? You might not be able to identify a single source of your weight gain and poor choices in diet, but the consequences are very real. It makes sense that as we age and our bodies become less active, the pounds begin to creep on. Decisions we have made in the past around what food we put in our bodies makes a difference now. We could get away with skimping on our diet or not exercising as frequently as we should. Now, dependent upon what we eat, our minds may not be as sharp, we may have frequent headaches, our body aches and it takes much longer to recuperate after working out. As we age, our metabolism slows down, so we can no longer eat the same quantities of food, or the high caloric, fatty foods we may have gotten away with when younger. We need to be more intentional about our health and recognize and understand that the choices we make have long-term ramifications.

No matter what your motivation for picking up this book, or your desire to regain some of that youthful energy, it's important to remember to revisit the reasons and use them as motivation. You may decide you want to have more energy to start each day, or to play with your children or grandchildren. You may want your clothes to fit better or have a special event you want to show up and dazzle. You may want to set a positive example for others – your children, grandchildren, peers, etc. Whatever the reasoning behind picking up this book, there are many ways you can incorporate small changes, today, this week and in this month that will have impact on your health. Your daily routine and what you choose to do today will shape the rest of the decisions you make about your future and becoming a fitter, healthier you.

It's important to start your morning off with nourishment and to wake your system up. The word breakfast is comprised of two words: Break which means to tear apart, to stop; and fast which in this context means to not eat. Breakfast then means to break the fast. When you wake up, it is likely your body has not had food for eight hours or more, causing the system to be in a state of relaxation and slowed down metabolism. It was conserving the energy you consumed for vital organs and similar operations. Try to make sure you have some protein and carbohydrate when you wake up. Depending upon your daily caloric requirements and your level of activity, you will need to consume between 300-675 calories at this meal.

If you are going to workout immediately after eating, determine what type of foods your body can handle and digest easily. Some items to consider may be oatmeal, cereal, orange juice, vegetable omelette, turkey bacon, and/or fruit. Some individuals cannot work out on a full stomach, so it may take time to understand and familiarize yourself with what your body is able to handle. I usually have cereal, milk and a banana before running, swimming or lifting. It works for me. If you are prone to upset stomachs, try something mild like a banana and oatmeal, a bagel with peanut butter or even yogurt. Power gels, power bars or smoothies are other options to consider and especially convenient. Get something in your system, and then make sure to replenish once you have finished your workout with something more substantial if needed. Carry around healthier food choices such as hummus and vegetables, almonds and raisins, apples, oranges or other pieces of fruit.

Let's explore ways you can incorporate more activity and movement into your already chaotic routine without detracting too much from what you deem to be essential. What often happens in life is that priorities start to push up against each other and they leave little room for individuals to identify health as a priority. So many believe it will be okay to just ignore, or because there is no "dire pressing need" it's on the back burner to revisit at a later date. More like, "I will get to that later," or "Someday I will…" It seems as though it is the one piece that can be tucked away and saved for later because there isn't a pressing immediate issue at hand…unlike the crying baby, the bills that need to get paid, the spouse that needs attention, the project that has a deadline in five hours, etc. If you can begin to look into the future and see the choices and decisions made today-or the inaction-and how they impact the quality of life and what you are able to do five, ten even twenty years from now, I can almost guarantee you would be changing some things right now and re-prioritizing.

What if the trajectory of your life as of this moment has you with high blood pressure, diabetes, heart failure, overweight and exhausted? These conditions can result in treatment costs of nearly $14,000 per year! When faced with a dollar amount, does it now seem to be more critical to make changes today? You can begin to combat these illnesses and costs by making changes TODAY. NOW is the time to start. This may seem a bit too simple, and you may be saying that will never work for me. The truth of the matter is, everybody is busy and can have a plethora of excuses as to why they don't fit fitness into their daily routine. It takes a small step in the right direction to get started, a belief in the value of making the changes, and a commitment to continue moving in that direction despite the setbacks—which will happen.

Rather than putting your health on the back burner, and trying to squeeze it in if you can, find the time and schedule it. Sometimes people want the support of others and to be held accountable. If this is you, schedule it with your friends. If the typical girls' night out is a movie and dinner, how about trying a walk and sampling healthy recipes at a friends' house? Try a new class, such as Pilates, yoga, Zumba or even pottery. You don't need to give up the camaraderie or what you enjoy. Schedule a session at the climbing wall instead of the margaritas. Grab some rackets and play tennis or badminton. Find your old self again and bring out the kid in you – go skating, bike riding or grab a ball and kick it around. If the guys always go for beer and watch the game, how about getting on the treadmills at your local health facility for the first half and watch on the monitors, then shower and catch the second half at the pub? You might still have some beer, but you will now be incorporating exercise into your day. Or grab a football to toss around, a frisbee to play ultimate frisbee or even take a bike ride to talk about the latest draft or trade.

If you feel like you need time to yourself to reflect and don't need someone working out with you, schedule your workout time as though it were a meeting. Everything else is on that to-do list and gets checked off, do this for your future self. You don't need to let others know what you are doing, but you need to make sure you have a time set aside for your health NOW.

Another way you can begin to incorporate health into your daily regime is every hour at work, do ten squats. By the end of the day you have done 80! Switch it up, do squats one hour, push-ups the next, sit-ups the next, jumping jacks, mountain climbers, plank exercises, etc. The idea is to make it simple for you to change, and incorporate into your already hectic schedule. Bring five pieces of fruit or servings of vegetables to work and put them on your desk each Monday. Make it a goal to have them finished by the end of the week. Instead of the chips you have throughout the day, bring pistachios, almonds or peanuts. Substitute fruit-infused water for your coffee, or Water Joe. It has the same amount of caffeine as a cup of coffee but it's water! If you usually take the bus to work, get off and on a stop early and walk the rest of the way. When you brush your teeth in the morning, add some squats, calf raises and side twists.

You have now added exercise into your schedule without inconveniencing yourself too much. If you drive, park as far away from your office, from the grocery store, mall entrance, church, down the block from your friend's house or restaurant, etc., as you can. Take the stairs instead of the elevator, at least for a couple floors. Before you know it, you will have started to lead a more active life and begun to eat healthier. By modifying little things, you will begin to notice a big difference by the end of the week, the month and definitely the year. You will have more energy, feel stronger, be more at peace and able to concentrate on tasks at hand.

You have begun to put your health at the forefront, congratulations.

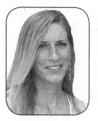

About Erika

Erika Binger is a former world triathlete and aquathlete champion. She has always been involved in some capacity with athletics and health. Growing up on a ranch provided a foundation in both of these areas, as she was often found working with the animals, climbing the hills, riding, working in the garden and spending time outdoors with her siblings. Growing up with fresh produce and meat was something she now feels incredibly blessed with, but at the time was normal. She believes, having grown up with these elements, that they contributed to the health she and her family still have today.

She started to be involved in sports during her middle school years and competed on her college basketball team her freshman year. After the first year, she decided to hang up her basketball shoes and donned a swimsuit instead. The swim coach had noticed her dedication and commitment outside of basketball practice and encouraged her to try the swim team, even though she had never swam competitively before. Binger went on to swim competitively for the remainder of her collegiate career and credits her swim coach with instilling one of her basic fundamentals she brings to her clients today –treat everyone fairly regardless of their experience and skill.

Upon graduation, Binger volunteered as a boy's basketball coach at a Boys and Girls Club, during which time she also rode her bike the length of the Mississippi River to raise funds for the programming. She was offered the Athletic Director's job, and during her career she developed and implemented a top-notch girls sports program – where prior to her involvement, there was none. At the same time, she grew the boys programming, and received several awards for her work. Simultaneously, she earned her Masters' Degree in Organizational Leadership and began to get her legs wet in triathlon. She competed nationally and internationally in the sport, with numerous podium finishes. After finishing an Ironman, she decided she did everything in the sport she set out to do, and since she didn't like biking, was going to focus on aquathlons.

She founded the V3 Youth Triathlon Team, which introduced and worked with many inner-city youth, in the sport of triathlon. Binger ensured the sport drew the athletes, but they would become top-notch individuals as well as athletes through the educational, goal-setting, nutritional, career and personal development aspects of the program. Several of her athletes have placed on the podium and the team won top honors at the national championships. In addition, every athlete that has completed the program is enrolled in college.

She also recognized the disconnect between spiritual and physical health, and was one of the founding members of her church's (Impact Living Christian Center) Health & Wellness Ministry. The H&WM now hosts an annual 5K to raise funds for college scholarships. She is currently pursuing another masters' degree in Nutrition and Exercise Physiology.

CHAPTER 17

ALL WE HAVE IS TIME

BY DOUG SCHLENK

I was nineteen years old and heading out on my first solo road trip from my home in St. Louis to Chicago to visit some friends. I was like every other nineteen year old in that I knew everything, so naturally this miniscule two hundred seventy miles would be a snap. I had been to Chicago before, but via train or as a passenger with my family for summer vacation. In both instances, I was too young to understand what you should pay attention to while driving. Since I had been driving for all of three years, this maiden voyage outside of the bi-state area did not concern me. My thoughts were focused on Chicago and the fun I was going to have, how I was going to get there was an afterthought.

This era of road travel was much different than how we travel today. The cell phone and GPS that we take for granted were not as easily accessible. The running joke at the time was that the only people that had access to cell phones were doctors and drug dealers. If you wanted directions to somewhere, you bought a map at a gas station. If you really needed to call someone while traveling, you would use a pay phone. So, here I am – no cell phone, no map - I was a nineteen year old know-it-all. Who needed a map? I get on the highway, go north, and follow the signs that say Chicago. According to my calculations I could go 80mph the entire way and be there in three-and-a-half to four hours tops.

My journey was as expected - beautiful flat cornfields, tractor trailers, and making great time. Then I hit the suburbs; who knew there would still be rush hour traffic on a Friday at seven o'clock in the evening. Come to find out this wasn't rush hour, it was known to the native residents as just traffic. It took nearly two and a half hours to finish the final forty miles into the city. Once into downtown, I was reenergized with excitement. The directions from my friends were so easy, get off the highway hang a couple lefts and rights, arrive, and let the party begin. Ninety minutes later and not recognizing anything that was described to me, panic began to set in. "Ok" I said to myself, "just find a place to park, walk to a pay phone, call, and find out where the hell I am at!" Find a place to park - If you are not familiar with Chicago, or any other downtown in a major city, there is no place to park.

Circling around the neighborhood, I notice a pay phone, "perfect now just a place to park." I took one more lap around the block, then I saw it as if there was a spotlight directing me to it, an open spot. How did I miss this the first five times I went by? Whatever, the spot was just off the street in a small parking lot and only half a block from the pay phone. I park, jog to the pay phone and make the call only to find out I was a couple hundred feet from my destination. "Yes!" I hustle back to my car, mind you the time elapsed from parking, to pay phone, make the call, and back to my car was less than five minutes. I turn the corner only to see my car being lifted up by a tow truck. My heart dropped into my stomach. This wasn't seriously happening, is it a car that looked like mine but it couldn't actually be mine, right? Wrong. So, I pleaded with the tow truck driver, "Hey, I am from out of town I didn't know I couldn't park there, I'm lost!" His reply, which I felt as though he had used it before, with a smile from ear to ear, "Welcome to Chicago, hope you have a nice visit!"

My perception prior to setting out on that journey was that it was going to be easy and quick. I had a start and a finish, but never took into consideration anything in between. I just knew where I wanted to go and used really bad information to try and get there. This is not that different to how you may perceive your body transformation goals. You know where you are and where you want to be. So, how

ALL WE HAVE IS TIME

do you get there? What map are you going to use? Once you have a map, which route are you going to take? Who will you call if you need better directions? What will you do when your car gets towed?

The fitness map I have developed over the years for the success of my clients has evolved, just as the map at the gas station is now a high tech GPS on your phone. These six steps will provide you with forethought and direction to planning and managing your time. Your fitness goals should become a part of your life and not take you from your life.

1.) Plan or You Plan to Fail

Sounds simple or at least it will become simple with practice. Each week should be looked at as a short trip from Sunday to Saturday. You must schedule your grocery shopping, food preparation, cooking, training, work, family and fun.

It is a lot to consider, but consider this: we all own the same 168 hours a week. Let's say work and commuting to work takes up 60 hours. Sleeping (if you get 8 hours) takes up another 56 hours, training for your goals 6 hours. That still leaves you with 46 hours a week for everything else. It's up to you to use these hours effectively, so your goals don't make you feel as if you are missing out on life. Take a look at your week as it is now, see what you can eliminate to give you more time for the things that truly matter.

"Exercise doesn't take time, it gives us time."

2.) Don't Shop till you Drop

Your trip to the grocery store should take less than 30 minutes. Yes, I am adding time for checkout. You say it can't be done, well it can, I do it every week shopping for my wife, two kids and myself.

Have your list of items made in the order in which you are going to encounter them in the store. This saves you time from either scanning up and down your list to see what other vegetables you need before you leave produce, and keeps you on a set course to keep from being distracted by things you do not need.

Second tip is stay out of the aisles. More time is wasted in the aisles with the mind numbing shelves of boxes and cans than anywhere else. Quite frankly, the foods you need for your goals won't be there anyway. Real foods don't have labels; those are the ones you want to eat a majority of the time anyway. If you can pick it, dig it, kill it then you should eat it. You want your food to be in its closest original form. Two items you will find in the aisles are spices and plastic storage containers, but this is a once every few months visit to restock.

3.) Cook in Bulk

You could have the greatest meal plan from the most renowned nutrition expert in the world. But if you think for a second, Wednesday night, after a hard day at work and the gym that you are going to fire up the grill and cook your chicken, boil some rice, and clean and cut your veggies, you are dead wrong.

This is where cooking enough food as if you are celebrating Thanksgiving will pay off. I have found even those who are experienced cooks get tired of putting in the effort that they normally would to create a fantastic meal every day. So, it's ok if you aren't an experienced cook, cooking in bulk will help you keep your nutrition on track. The easiest tool for cooking in bulk is the slow cooker or crock pot. Meat, spices, turn ON, and leave it alone for 4-8 hours. Go to work and come home to a house that smells like your mom has been there all day cooking. I think most can handle those complicated instructions. Go online and order a healthy eating crock pot recipes book and now you don't have to create your own dishes. Make sure to cook enough to give you your protein source for at least 3 days of meals.

Now even though you have been eating your whole life, cooking in bulk will take some trial and error to master. But eventually it will save you time and the guilt of ordering pizza on Wednesday night.

4.) Your Training must be Meaningful

The old adage "something is better than nothing," does not apply here. I often have found that those who train with this attitude never reach their potential and inevitably fail. Just as you must plan your grocery list, your workout must also be detailed. If you show up to the gym and don't have a starting or finishing point you will be repeating the aforementioned phrase.

If you are not supremely confident on designing a program for your goals, then hire someone. Don't buy a magazine and use whatever workout they are offering this month. To this day, I pay for help whether it's with my training or my business, there is always someone who knows more and will help get you out of your norm.

So, now you have a routine, you know how much time you have to complete the workout, now you must OWN IT! Your focus has to be on the task at hand. All other distractions are left outside, this time is yours, remember why you started the journey and what it will take to get to your destination. You don't need to check the Facebook status of your "ex"; the only status you need to know is how much weight and how many reps.

5.) Know your Social Schedule

This is the tow truck driver that will smile and tell you to have a nice visit. The lack of planning for social events may be the most overlooked aspect of one's life when trying to achieve a transformation goal. You are a human being, not a machine; we find emotional comfort when gathering with friends and family over food and drink. In order to enjoy the event and not get towed away from your goals we have to, wait for it, plan. You know when your social event will take place, and probably what will be served. I know this isn't sexy but if you are perfect with your training and eating leading up to the event, then about an hour prior to, have a filling snack or small meal. You won't end up parked in a tow away zone next to a table unconsciously eating and drinking 1000 empty calories due to hunger.

Nonetheless, you were invited to a social event. So, take part in food and drink, in light moderation. Just as long as you don't overindulge and get back on path the next day, you will continue to your destination no worse for wear.

6.) K.I.S.S.

Depending on your personality, the above acronym could mean two things. Keep it simple stupid/silly; I have a tendency to be hard on myself so I prefer the first option. Regardless of which you prefer, this final step is a reminder not to overthink the process. You are capable of anything you commit to wholeheartedly. But the commitment must be internalized within you. You have to believe in yourself. The only thing that can hold you back is you. So, K.I.S.S. – develop your map to your goals, follow it regardless of what detours may slow you down. Trust me, there will be detours, but as long as you have a map, you will find your way back on course to complete your journey.

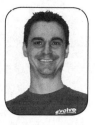

About Doug

Douglas Schlenk helps everyday people achieve extraordinary results. Being raised by active parents, especially by a father with an extensive athletic and coaching background, he naturally gravitated towards athletics and fitness. Doug's interest in strength training began in high school, and while trying to improve his own athletic performance, he purchased his first fitness book. In the years to come, he would continue to self-educate through books, seminars, and networking with coaches. But, it still took working five years in Corporate America before he realized his true calling to help people better their own lives.

Doug's training philosophy is "to stimulate not annihilate his clients." His goal with each client is to make them better at the activities that they enjoy doing – whether they are a weekend warrior or just want to be able to play with their kids or grandkids. Doug and his team of coaches help people realize that they can achieve their goals without sacrificing time from the things that truly matter.

Doug has been coaching people for 12 years and has established his own training facility, Evolve Personal Fitness, over the last 5 years. Doug has been featured on the local T.V. news outlets with success stories of his clients and the time-saving training methods that he uses. He has also been selected as one of America's Premier Experts and has been featured in the St. Louis Post Dispatch's Health section. Doug and his team are active in the community – holding charity classes each month to raise money for local charities, and donating their time and knowledge speaking to local businesses about exercise and nutrition.

You can connect with Doug at:
dms_fitness@yahoo.com
www.evolvepersonalfit.com
www.faccbook.com/douglas.schlenk

CHAPTER 18

SIX SIMPLE STEPS TO SEXY ABS

BY GINA VIEGAS, MSC

Imagine waking up every morning loving what you see in the mirror. No need for an alarm-clock, you jump out of bed feeling energised and confident. What's more, you've got the body of your dreams. Can you sense how that would feel?

If this sounds like a distant dream, it's time to take action. I'm going to reveal six simple but powerfully effective steps you can start to take right now, which will lead to flat and sexy abs. The truth is, you can have your ultimate dream body. Keep reading, because I'm about to share every detail of how I got my sexy stomach, so you can too.

You've invested in this book called *Rapid Body Makeover*, so I'm assuming you want to transform your body, fast. You're not alone! I'm a busy coach at a boutique fitness studio in London's Canary Wharf, where my clients are some of the most successful people in the City. Yet they all share one concern. When I ask a new client about the body part they want to transform as soon as possible, top of the list is…their abs.

Call it a washboard stomach, a six-pack or abs of steel, we all understand the language of a flat, strong and lean stomach. Great abs are a badge of honour for people like you who take health and fitness seriously. After all, nothing shouts sexy body louder than sexy abs, right? And sexy abs are about more than just aesthetics. A flat and lean midsection tells the world that you're a focused, dedicated individual who is in great health thanks to the choices you make every day.

A body makeover is about transformation and transition. It offers the ultimate possibility: to reinvent yourself. That is exactly what I did, and it's why I have so much success working as a wellness coach and body transformation expert. I grew up eating healthy, homemade food and never had problems with my weight. That all started to change when I moved from Portugal to the UK. I started working in the high-pressure environment of London's financial sector at age 23. It's a familiar story: I was stressed, working long hours, not doing enough exercise and making poor food choices. I was tired and frustrated with my ever-growing waistline. I just couldn't work out how to shift the fat.

After years of failed diets, unused gym memberships and too much "starting over", I finally decided to seek professional help. It was the best decision I ever made. My body transformation began when I employed a nutritionist and a personal trainer. And my life changed along with my physique! I became fascinated with understanding how food and exercise impacted my body, and realised I had to help other people achieve the same success. I decided to change careers and become an educator and coach in health and wellness. And, yes, I got my flat stomach.

Here's a shocking bit of history about our waistlines. In the 1950s, the average waist measurement for adult women was 28". Fast-forward to 2012 and the average was 34". Men haven't fared much better: the average man's waist these days is 37". Declining activity levels, high ongoing stress, and growing portion sizes are just some of the reasons behind our expanding waistlines.

What does it take to reveal a sexy six-pack? It's not just about toning up the abdominal muscles. We also need to reduce body fat levels sufficiently so we can show off the definition: after all, there's no point having your six-pack hidden under a layer of fat! And it's important to manage stress and key hormones.

There are six steps you simply must take if you ever hope to have a flat, firm, lean and sexy stomach:

ONE: DEFINE AND RECORD YOUR GOAL

Goal-setting is one of the first things I tackle when coaching new clients. Vague goals just won't cut it. To be successful in life (particularly your body transformation), you need to be super clear about the details. Set SMART goals: specific, measurable, achievable, relevant and time-based.

S – A **Specific** goal is clearly defined. Rather than saying "I want a flat stomach," be more specific: How many inches do you want your waist to be, or what body fat percentage do you want to reach?

M – A **Measurable** goal can be quantified. This is important so that you can track your results as you go along, and so you know when you've reached them!

A – **Achievable** goals can still be challenging and certainly doable with hard work and dedication. Choose a goal which is tough enough to excite you, but achievable with the correct tools, techniques and coaching support.

R – Set **Realistic** goals that aren't small, lazy or easy. Settle for a goal which is too small and you will quickly lose motivation. Instead, set a goal which gets you fired up and ready to take massive action every single day.

T – **Time-based** goal setting will help you achieve your target. Use a specific date, like a holiday, birthday or photoshoot, so you can put your goal in your calendar and count down to it. No moving the goal posts!

Write your goal down in the present tense, as if you have already achieved it. Dig deep into the details. How do you feel? What are you doing now you've got flat abs? What type of clothes do you wear? How do people react to the new you, what do they say? How does it feel to run your hands over your flat abs and around your toned waist? Put your written goals somewhere you'll see them every morning and evening. This will really help you stay motivated and on track.

When I wanted to get my sexy abs back, I set a very specific goal that included a waist measurement (I based it on the waist measurement of a celebrity whose shape was similar to mine and whose physique I aspired to). Knowing that my waist was going to look like hers kept my motivation fired up!

TWO: GET A HANDLE ON HEALTHY NUTRITION

You often hear health professionals saying that diets don't work. Actually, they do. The trouble strikes when it comes to maintenance. Research shows that only 5% of dieters are successful in maintaining their shape. In fact, 95% regain any fat loss within five years.

Why does this happen, and how can you be one of the 5%? Successful fat loss comes from making positive changes to eating habits for life. When people are on a "diet", they can't wait for it to end so they can go back to "eating normally". The trouble is, that "normal eating" is what caused them to get out of shape in the first place.

Approach your nutrition in two phases: body transformation, and maintenance. Start as you mean to go on, by choosing a sustainable nutrition plan that you feel you can follow in the long term. Eat carbohydrates low on the glycemic index (GI): avoid white bread, boxed cereals, white potatoes and junk food like pizzas (high GI) and opt for leafy vegetables, berries and oranges (low GI). Get several servings of vegetables and leafy greens, plenty of protein, and healthy fats such as olive oil, nuts, avocados and oily fish. Eliminate all grains, processed sugars and sweeteners, including those in drinks.

To maintain, eat in a similar way to your body transformation phase, but slowly add higher glycemic vegetables and some fruit, plenty of healthy fats and occasionally some of your favorite foods which contain grains. Aim for that happy 80-20 rule and eat healthily at least 80% of the time.

THREE: EXERCISE SMARTER AND HARDER,

NOT LONGER

Latest research shows that shorter, more intense exercise sessions based around weight training is actually more effective than longer sessions of slow-paced cardio. Make interval training and resistance work the mainstay of your exercise sessions. Training too frequently, not getting adequate rest, and doing long sessions of cardiovascular work will actually over-stress your body, encouraging it to produce stress hormones such as cortisol (which slam the brakes on abdominal fat loss).

Do 20-minute sessions of intense interval work to torch calories from body fat, and keep your metabolism high for hours. Weight training will keep your lean mass high as you lose fat, resulting in a tight waistline.

FOUR: BALANCE YOUR HORMONES

Did you ever consider that hormones play a huge role in getting sexy abs? Keep your hormones happy, and your body will be more willing to play ball.

We're not just talking about the sex hormones testosterone and oestrogen. Knowledge of the master hormones including insulin, cortisol and Human Growth Hormone will give you the edge over everyone else.

Insulin, the fat-storage hormone, is produced by the pancreas when we consume high GI carbohydrates and shuttles the sugars into cells. The trouble is, most of us don't need that much-stored energy. So, what happens to the sugars? They get stored as body fat. To lose body fat, we need to convince our body's energy systems to consume stored fat as fuel. This process begins when we deny the body its favorite energy source: glucose (blood sugar).

Cortisol, the stress hormone, becomes troublesome when it's released in large quantities over a prolonged period of time. If you're constantly feeling overwhelmed, exhausted and stressed, your body is producing more cortisol than it can cope with. Long periods of exercise, particularly cardio, are interpreted by the body as yet another stress, only adding to the problem. Excess cortisol prevents optimal muscle tissue growth and encourages the conversion of protein into glucose. The result is fat storage, particularly around your belly. Not great when your goal is sexy, defined abs.

Human Growth Hormone (HGH) governs muscle size and bone strength, the size of our internal organs, cell health and tissue repair. From the age of 30, production declines rapidly, so optimising HGH is essential for getting into shape. The great news is that exercise is the largest single contributor to boosting HGH release. Studies have shown that high intensity intervals on a stationary bike increase HGH secretion by 166%, but weight training resistance at maximal lift capacity increases it by 400%! Just one more reason to strength train for sexy abs.

FIVE: GET A GREAT COACH

There are so many benefits of working with a fat loss coach:

- You'll get direct access to scientifically-based, research-proven techniques and protocols without wasting time on trial and error.

- Your coach will be able to track your progress using industry techniques such as caliper skinfold tests and body fat tests.

- You'll have a dedicated fat-loss professional supporting you, encouraging you and motivating you even when you want to give up.

- Your coach will give you a form of accountability, helping you stick to your goals and move forward every single day.

- You'll get value-added extras like fitness industry updates, latest research news and access to cutting-edge techniques.

It's really important to choose the right coach. Don't be afraid to ask questions, seek testimonials and go with your gut feeling before you invest. This is going to be one of the most important relationships you'll ever make. It can truly change your life.

SIX: TRACK YOUR EFFORTS TO VALUE

THE RESULTS

I've already said that the most successful goals are measurable. So make sure you measure yours as you progress through this fantastic journey to sexy abs. You could keep a paper or online journal, a personal blog or use mobile apps to track data. The key is consistency. Here are some valuable data points to note:

- workouts (date, duration, content)
- nutrition (macronutrient balance, ingredient choices, timings, frequency)
- sleep (timing and quality)
- feelings (energy, mood, fatigue)
- measurements (weight, body fat, waist measurement, photos)

Tracking will keep you on course as you close in on your goal and will provide you with an incredible resource. Data is a goldmine of information. Yours will become the basis of your very own flat abs blueprint for life.

You're about to embark on an amazing journey of self-discovery and body transformation. Make it a story you can look back on with pride!

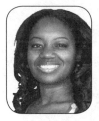

About Gina

Gina Viegas, MSc is a Body Transformation Expert and Wellness Coach who has been involved in helping hundreds of people get into great shape and health. She has been featured in local, national and international media. Gina's programmes and no-nonsense approach to health and fitness help busy people strip away unwanted body fat and reach their ultimate dream body. She is passionate about helping people reach their health and fitness goals and seeing the boost in confidence it subsequently gives them across many areas of their lives.

Originally from Portugal, Gina moved to the United Kingdom when she was 22 to do a Master's degree in Business and Management. After her degree, she moved to London and has been living there ever since. Gina's background in the financial world gives her a good insight into the pressures of executive life. Long hours, lack of exercise, poor nutrition and high stress levels were a dangerous combination that caused Gina to become overweight, frustrated and unable to enjoy the type of vibrant life she used to lead. She decided to transform her body and life. She studied fitness, holistic nutrition, NLP and humanistic psychology to arm her with the skills that helped her to transform her shape (she lost 60lbs of fat) and her life. This inspired her to become a wellness coach.

Gina offers Wellness Coaching in person and online to clients all over the world. She also owns a boutique personal training studio in the heart of London's financial district, specialising in rapid fat loss and lifelong maintenance programs for everyone from CEOs to actors to busy mothers.

Gina is constantly studying the latest research in exercise, nutrition and personal development to help improve her clients' health, wellness and general wellbeing. She is a published author and a speaker on the topics of holistic nutrition, fitness, wellness and weight loss.

For more information about Gina, visit: www.ginaviegas.com
Email: info@ginaviegas.com